Harry
Warm
& best
Beverly J. Capock

Other monographs in the series, *Major Problems in Clinical Surgery:*

Jackman and Beahrs: *Tumors of the Large Bowel*—to be published 1968

Haller: *Deep Thrombophlebitis*

Spratt and Donegan: *Cancer of the Breast*

Barker: *Peripheral Arterial Disease*

Madding and Kennedy: *Trauma to the Liver*

Welch: *Polypoid Lesions of the Gastrointestinal Tract*

Child et al.: *The Liver and Portal Hypertension*

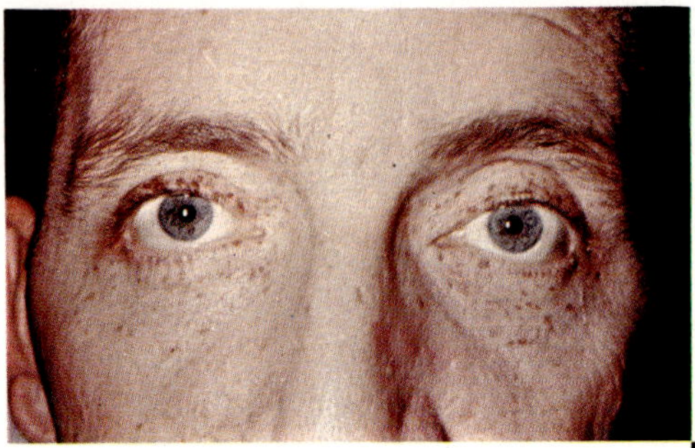

A. Peutz-Jeghers syndrome pigmentation.

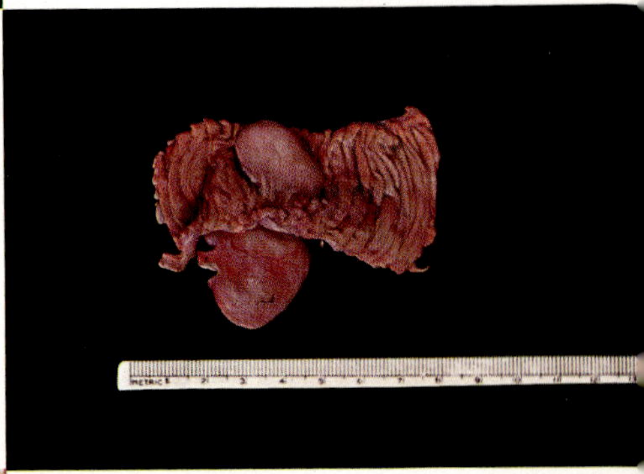

B. Submucosal leiomyoma and diverticulum of jejunum.

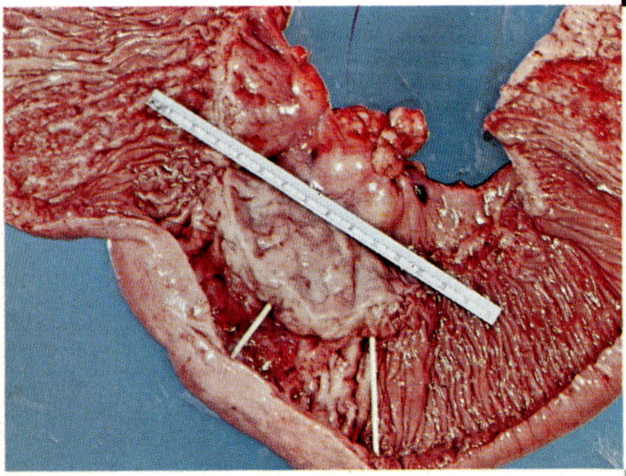

C. Lymphocytoma of ileum.

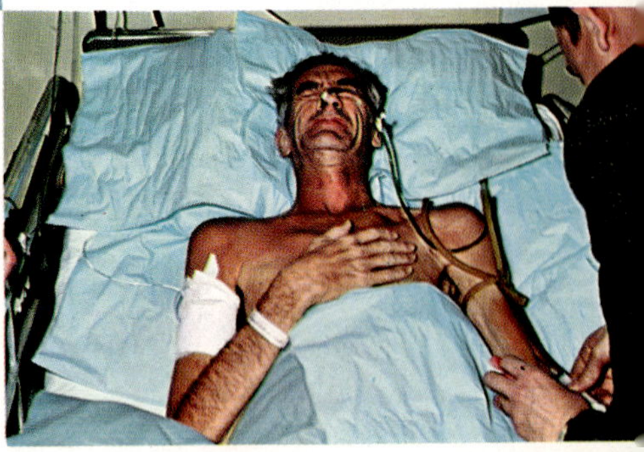

D. Onset of carcinoid flush (neck and upper thorax).

SURGERY OF THE SMALL INTESTINE IN THE ADULT

by

Bentley P. Colcock, M.D.

and

John W. Braasch, M.D.

Department of Surgery,
Lahey Clinic Foundation,
Boston, Massachusetts

Volume VII in the Series

MAJOR PROBLEMS IN CLINICAL SURGERY

J. ENGLEBERT DUNPHY, M.D.
Consulting Editor

W. B. Saunders Company, Philadelphia, London, Toronto, 1968

W. B. Saunders Company: West Washington Square
Philadelphia, Pa. 19105

12 Dyott Street
London W.C.1

1835 Yonge Street
Toronto 7, Ontario

Surgery of the Small Intestine in the Adult

 Library of Congress catalog card number 67-25735.

Dedicated To

RICHARD BARTLEY CATTELL, M.D.

1900–1964

Master Surgeon

Foreword

The need for surgical operations on the small bowel has increased considerably in recent years. Chronic vascular insufficiency, acute mesenteric vascular occlusion, the blind loop syndrome, fistulas, and neoplasms, formerly regarded as rare indications, have become comparatively common. Improved management of acute intestinal obstruction, newer concepts of the place of surgery in regional ileitis and the superior mesenteric artery syndrome, as well as the use of small bowel procedures in the treatment of obesity, on the one hand, and malnutrition on the other, make it essential for the general surgeon to have a thorough understanding of the principles of small bowel surgery.

In this volume Doctors Colcock and Braasch have made available for the practicing surgeon an up-to-date presentation of all the important aspects of modern small bowel surgery.

J. Englebert Dunphy

Preface

Interest in the small intestine—and in its surgical diseases—has long been eclipsed by its near neighbors, the stomach and colon. We must recognize, however, that the small bowel is the most common site of gastrointestinal obstruction. Furthermore, small intestinal insufficiency, small bowel carcinoid tumors, mesenteric vascular insufficiency, nonpeptic ulcers, diverticular disease, and inflammatory disease of the small intestine have assumed an increasing importance in the surgical literature of recent times. We have attempted in this work to survey and coordinate current thinking and background material on all surgical disease of the adult small intestine and to integrate this with our considerable experience in these areas. To our knowledge, there is no other single source of this information available.

Our thanks for help in preparing this monograph go to Doctors Warren Nickerson, Claude Fortin, John Vansant, Alan Hume, Howard Denbo, and Clifford Chang, former residents in surgery at the Lahey Clinic Foundation. Our special appreciation is extended to Mr. P. D. Malone and Mr. Frank Steckel for art work, to Mr. George Buchanan for photographic illustrations, and to Mrs. Nancy Braasch, Mrs. Ruth Keddy, and Miss Charlotte Thompson for editorial assistance.

THE AUTHORS

Contents

Chapter One

ANATOMY

LENGTH

It is surprising that such a simple measurement as the length of the small intestine should not be generally known since its practical application to resective procedures and the short bowel syndrome is so important. Most estimations of the length of the small intestine are made in the postmortem room or anatomy laboratory after removal of the mesentery, which allows considerable elongation of the bowel. Such measurements are usually about 22 feet; Treves[7] mentioned extremes of $15\frac{1}{2}$ and $31\frac{1}{2}$ feet.

Exact measurements of the length of the combined jejunum and ileum are difficult at laparotomy because of the obvious elasticity of the tissues involved. The mean length in situ of these two portions of the small intestine is most often estimated at 9 or 10 feet.[1] The duodenum is approximately 10 inches in length, either in situ or after removal from the body.

DUODENUM

The duodenum is divisible into four parts (Fig. 1–1). The first or superior portion is almost 2 inches in length, begins at the pylorus, and ends at the neck of the gallbladder, where it makes an abrupt descent. In profile it is cone-shaped, and it is covered by peritoneum for most of its extent except for its posterior portion. Its anterior relationship is often with the gall-bladder or quadrate lobe of the liver; posteriorly it is contiguous with the gastroduodenal artery, the common bile duct, and the portal vein; and below and behind it is adjacent to the head and neck of the pancreas.

The second portion of the duodenum is about $3\frac{1}{2}$ inches in length and proceeds caudally from the first lumbar vertebra almost to the fourth.

It is covered by peritoneum anteriorly and overlies the spermatic or ovarian vein and the vena cava posteriorly and, variably, the hilus of the right kidney. Its inferior portion is covered by the peritoneum and vessels of the transverse mesocolon. Medially its convexity enfolds the head of the pancreas and is pierced by the termination of the common bile duct and the main and accessory pancreatic ducts.

The horizontal or third portion of the duodenum is approximately $2\frac{1}{2}$ inches in length and passes from right to left with some cephalad inclination over the upper border of the fourth lumbar vertebra. In so doing it passes over the vena cava and aorta, after which it terminates in the fourth portion. As it crosses the aorta, it in turn is crossed by the superior mesenteric vessels as they arise from their parent vessels and descend to the intestine. Superiorly, this portion of the duodenum is in relationship to the pancreas.

The ascending (fourth) portion of the duodenum measures about 1 inch in length and ascends as far as the upper border of the second lumbar vertebra, where it swings anteriorly to become the jejunum. This duodenojejunal flexure is suspended in the abdomen by a fibrous band, the ligament of Treitz, which in turn is attached to the connective tissue around the celiac artery and left crus of the diaphragm. The fourth portion of the duodenum is related posteriorly to the left psoas major muscle and left renal vessels.

It is then seen that the duodenum forms a C shape which clutches the head of the pancreas and is a fixed retroperitoneal organ covered in part by the mesocolon, stomach, colon, and gastrocolic omentum.

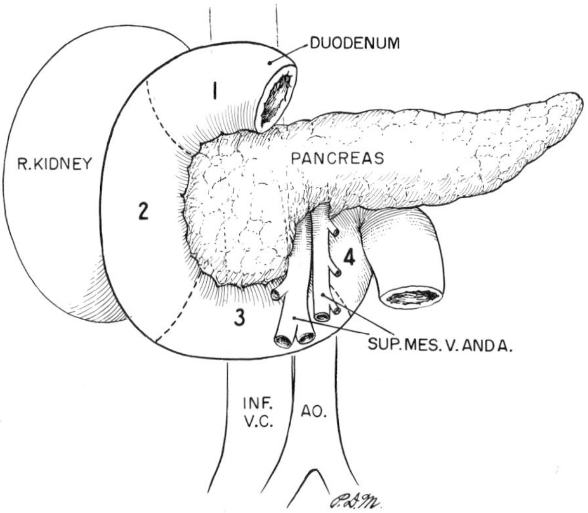

Figure 1–1. Divisions and relationships of the duodenum.

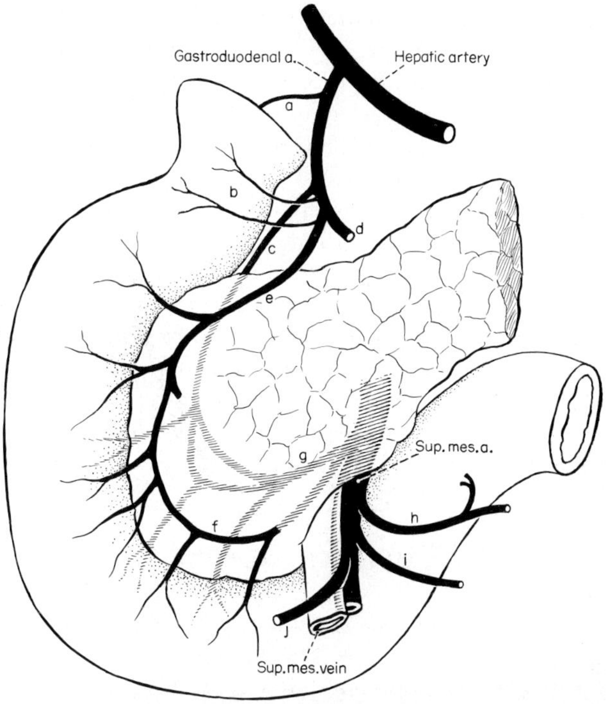

Figure 1–2. Arterial blood supply to duodenum. *a,* Posterior duodenal artery; *b,* anterior duodenal arteries; *c,* posterior superior pancreaticoduodenal artery; *d,* right gastroepiploic artery; *e,* anterior superior pancreaticoduodenal artery; *f,* anterior inferior pancreaticoduodenal artery; *g,* posterior inferior pancreaticoduodenal artery; *h,* duodenojejunal artery; *i,* jejunal artery; *j,* middle colic artery. (Adapted from Hollinshead, W. H.: Anatomy for Surgeons. New York, Paul B. Hoeber, Inc., 1956, p. 421.)

The arterial blood supply to the duodenum is derived from the hepatic and superior mesenteric arteries through the gastroduodenal, anterior, and posterior duodenal arteries and through the superior pancreaticoduodenal and inferior pancreaticoduodenal arteries, which anastomose to form an enmeshing network (Fig. 1–2). The venous supply is variable and drains into the splenic, superior mesenteric, and portal veins.

JEJUNUM AND ILEUM

The jejunum and ileum constitute the remainder of the small intestine and terminate in the right lower quadrant at a juncture with the cecum at the ileocecal valve. Proportionately the jejunum accounts for about two fifths of this combined length with the ileum making up three fifths. The loops of jejunum are usually found in the left portion of the abdomen and those of the ileum in the pelvis and right lower quadrant.

The duodenum (except the proximal portion), jejunum, and ileum present on their mucosal surfaces circular folds called valvulae conniventes or valves of Kerckring. These are made up of mucosal and submucosal layers with a firm connective tissue core. The majority of these folds extend for about two thirds of the circumference of the bowel cylinder and are visible on plain abdominal films of patients with obstruction.

The jejunum and ileum are supplied by the superior mesenteric artery and vein, which form the substance of the mesentery to the free small bowel. This mesentery is fan-shaped with a narrow 6-inch base attached to the posterior abdominal wall along a line down the posterior parietes from left to right from the body of the second lumbar vertebra to the sacroiliac articulation on the right. This mesentery contains blood vessels, lymphatics (lacteals), lymph nodes, nerves, and a variable amount of fat.

LYMPHATIC SUPPLY

The lymphatic supply of the small bowel is composed of the collecting vessels in the intestinal wall and mesentery, and the lacteals which follow the arterial and venous supply draining into the mesenteric nodes and eventually into the preaortic nodes. The lymphatic vessels of the duodenum drain into an anterior and posterior set situated along the pancreatico-duodenal groove. From these nodes, drainage is superiorly to those along the hepatic artery, to the subpyloric position, and inferiorly to those around the first portion of the superior mesenteric artery.

NERVE SUPPLY

The small intestine receives its nerve supply through the autonomic nervous system, which includes both afferent and efferent fibers. The latter (efferent) are both sympathetic and parasympathetic in distribution and function. Structurally the vagus nerve carries parasympathetic fibers to the small bowel via the posterior or right vagus nerve and the celiac and superior mesenteric plexus. In addition, the vagus nerve might also be a conveyor of afferent impulses. The sympathetic fibers reach the small intestine via the lesser and greater splanchnic nerves and the celiac and superior mesenteric plexuses. From these plexuses the fibers follow the superior mesenteric vessels to the bowel wall. The sympathetic fibers synapse in the abdominal ganglia from whence postganglionic fibers travel to the bowel. The parasympathetic fibers do not synapse until the plexuses of Auerbach and Meissner are reached between the circular and longitudinal muscle layers of the bowel wall and in the submucosal layer respectively.

APPLIED ANATOMY OF SMALL INTESTINE

The relationships of the junction of the second and the third portions of the duodenum to the mesentery of the transverse colon and to the head of the pancreas and vena cava are shown in Figures 1–3 and 1–4. These relationships are of importance in accomplishing Kocher's maneuver, basic to operative procedures on the duodenum and the termination of the biliary and pancreatic ducts. Note in Figure 1–3 the beginning of the dissection for the elevation of the second portion of the duodenum. This dissection stays close to the bowel wall and begins at the most inferior portion of the duodenum that is accessible before it becomes covered by the mesentery of the colon. It is necessary to use sharp dissection only over a short 2 or 3 cm. segment, since finger dissection safely completes the maneuver from right to left over the aorta and superiorly until the whole head and neck of the pancreas is in the palm of the operator's hand. Following this maneuver, the right lateral attachments of the duodenum can be severed, frequently without clamping vessels. Figure 1–4 demonstrates the exposure of the second portion of the duodenum gained by the completed Kocher maneuver and the relationships of the duodenum to adjacent structures.

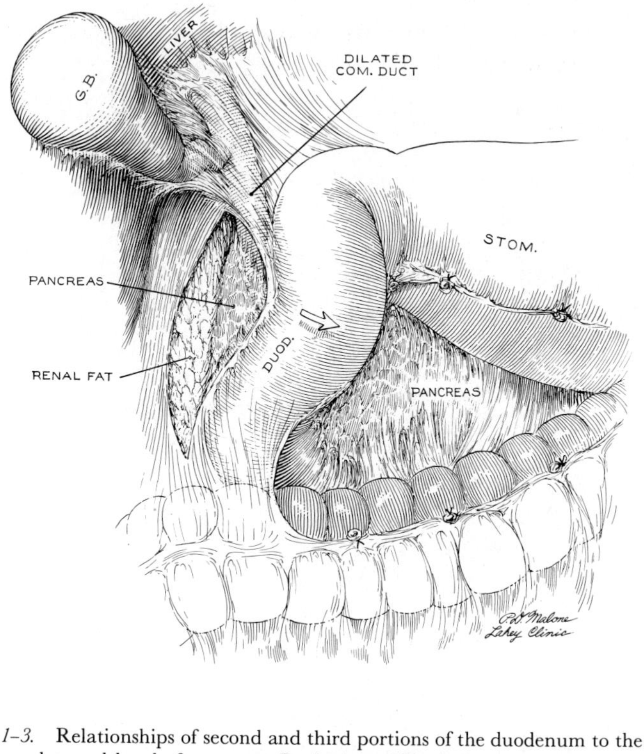

Figure 1–3. Relationships of second and third portions of the duodenum to the mesentery of transverse colon and head of pancreas. Beginning of Kocher's maneuver.

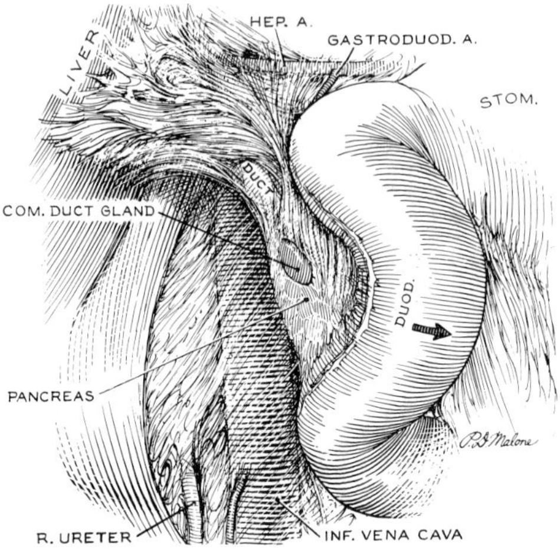

Figure 1–4. Relationships of second and third portions of the duodenum to the vena cava, spermatic vein, common bile duct, and common duct gland. Last dissection to elevate completely the second portion of the duodenum.

Figure 1–5 depicts a lateral view of the third portion of the duodenum as it passes from right to left between the aorta posteriorly and the superior mesenteric vessels anteriorly. Dilatation of the proximal duodenum with slow emptying of this portion has been ascribed to obstruction at this point by the mesenteric vessels occluding the bowel against the aorta.

The blood supply to the first portion of the jejunum is of extreme importance in pancreaticoduodenal resection or in other procedures involv-

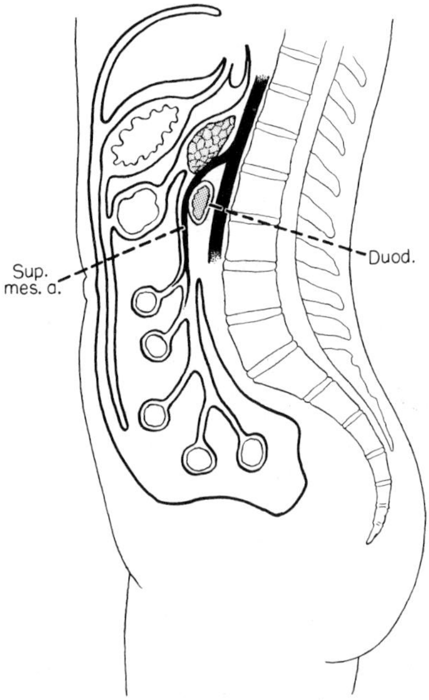

Figure 1–5. Lateral view of the third portion of the duodenum in its location between the superior mesenteric vessels anteriorly and the aorta posteriorly.

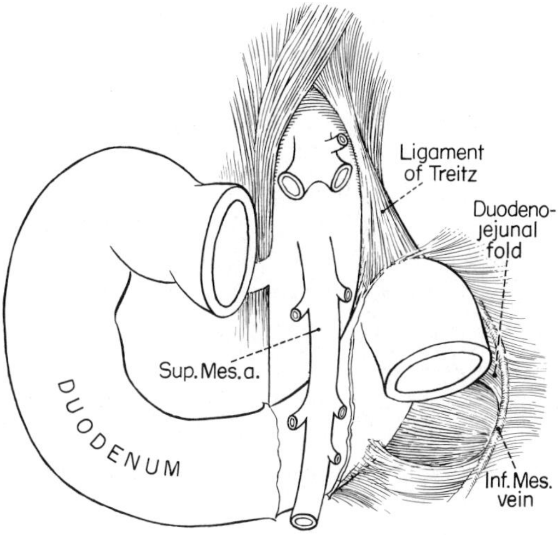

Figure 1–6. Ligaments and folds of the duodenojejunal flexure.

ing this portion of the small intestine. Figure 1–2 shows the first branches of the superior mesenteric artery to be jejunal branches that do not anastomose freely with each other and are very short. Extreme care must be exercised in resecting this portion of the jejunum and the duodenojejunal flexure so as not to compromise the blood supply, especially to the proximal segment.

Figure 1–6 shows the duodenojejunal flexure attached superiorly to the left diaphragmatic crus by the ligament of Treitz and laterally by the

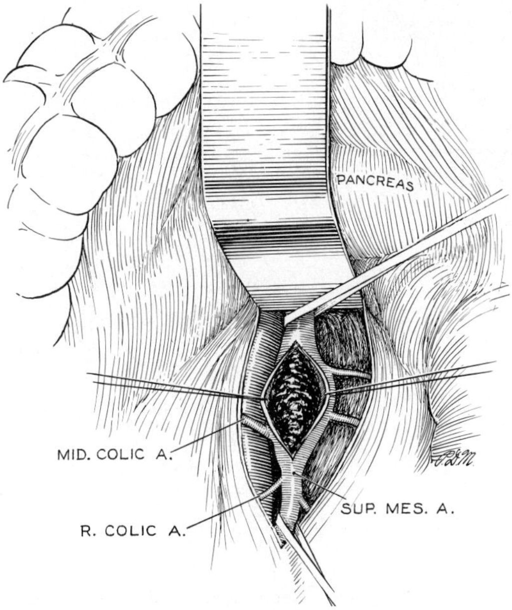

Figure 1–7. Position and branches of superior mesenteric artery relative to occlusion of this artery.

duodenojejunal fold. These ligaments may vary in length, breadth, and site of attachment to the duodenojejunal flexure; they are of importance in procedures involving the first portion of the jejunum, as essential length of bowel may be obtained by sectioning them over to the superior mesenteric vessels.

Figure 1–7 illustrates the first portion of the superior mesenteric artery and its branches. In the surgical treatment of occlusion of the superior mesenteric artery by embolus or thrombus, exposure of this region is essential. In this regard the following points are worth noting. First, the origin of the superior mesenteric artery is usually under the neck or body of the pancreas. The origin is thus rather inaccessible to direct anterior approach, as is the aorta in this region. Second, emboli to the superior mesenteric artery ordinarily lodge at a point of sudden narrowing, usually just after the middle colic artery has been given off. Thus, the artery is more

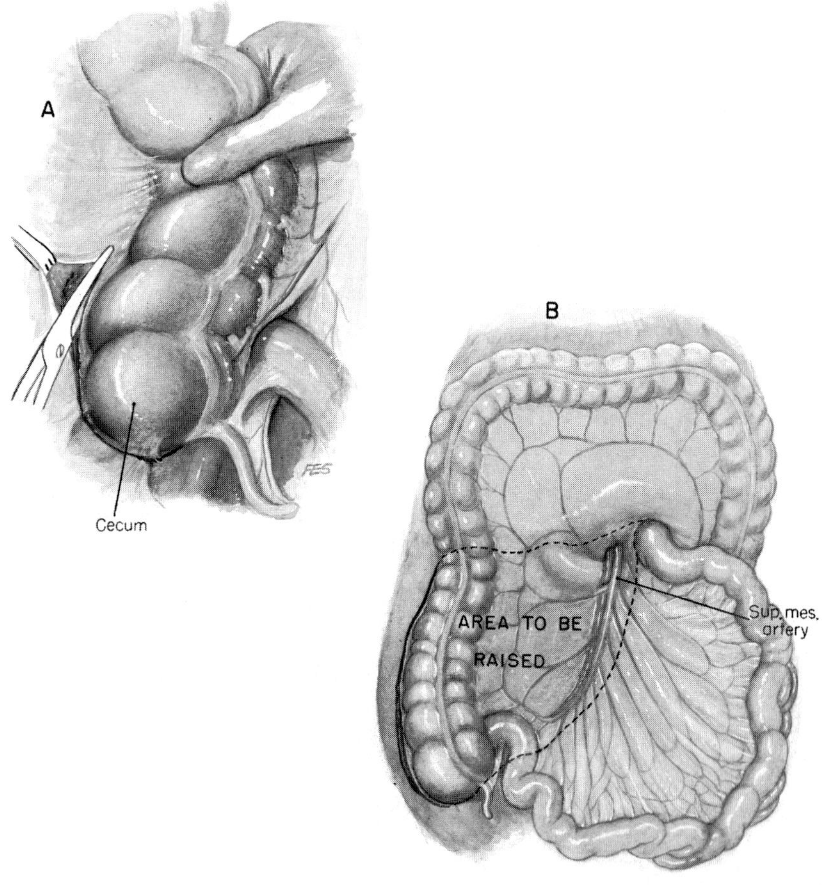

Figure 1–8. Exposure of third and fourth portions of the duodenum. Initial dissection for mobilization of the right side of the colon, small intestine, and mesentery is shown in *A*. (From Cattell, R. B., and Braasch, J. W.: Surg. Gynec. & Obst. *111*:378, 1960.)

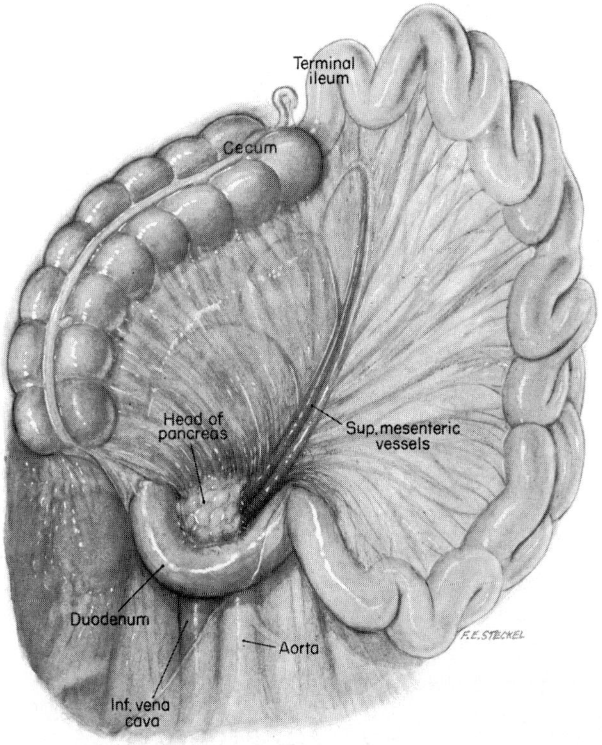

Figure 1–9. Exposure obtained of the third and fourth portions of the duodenum. (From Cattell, R. B., and Braasch, J. W.: Surg. Gynec. & Obst. *111*:378, 1960.)

readily accessible for dealing directly with embolic occlusion than for endarterectomy of the superior mesenteric artery takeoff.

The method of surgical exposure of the third and fourth portions of the duodenum is shown in Figures 1–8 and 1–9.[3] Since the mesentery of the right colon and small intestine is fused in uterine life with the posterior parietes, a line of cleavage exists which can be dissected to raise these organs and give direct access to the retroperitoneal duodenum.

Identification of a specific segment of small intestine is at times of enormous importance. Figure 1–10 and Table 1–1 indicate the differences between proximal jejunum and distal ileum. Note that the blood supply to these segments differs since the vessels to the ileum form many more arcades than those to the jejunum. The wall of the jejunum is much thicker than that of the ileum, the mesenteric fat in the ileum "creeps" up over the bowel wall for a short distance, the lumen in the ileum is smaller than in the jejunum, and the valvulae conniventes are much less marked in the ileum than in the jejunum.

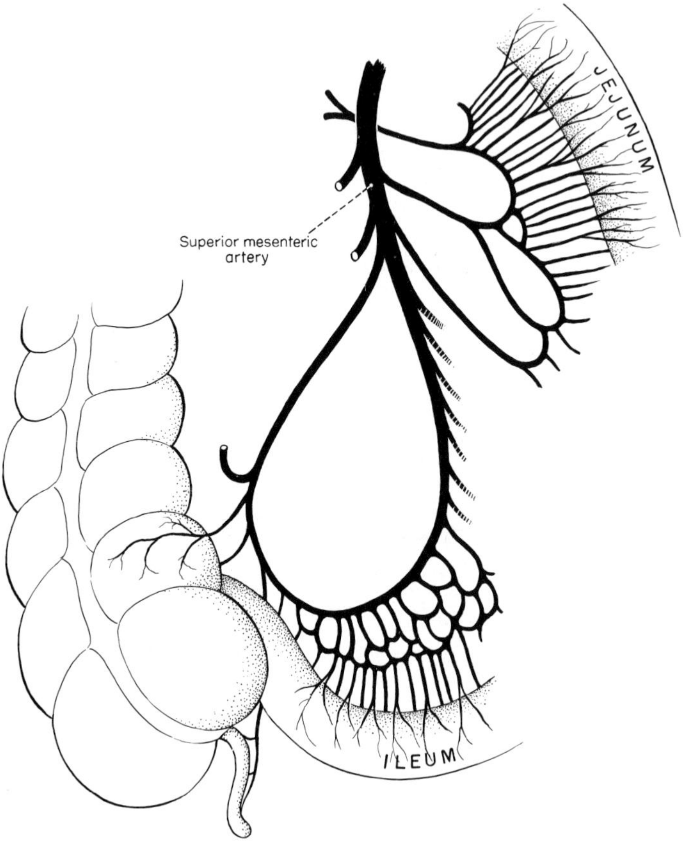

Figure 1–10. Blood supply to the jejunum and ileum. Note difference in arcades. (Adapted from Hollinshead, W. H.: Anatomy for Surgeons. New York, Paul B. Hoeber, Inc., 1956, p. 472.)

Table 1–1. Gross Differences Between Jejunum and Ileum

	JEJUNUM	ILEUM
Wall	Thick	Thin
Lumen	Large	Smaller
Mesenteric fat	On mesentery	On bowel and mesentery
Valvulae conniventes	Prominent	Less prominent
Blood supply	Single arcades	Several arcades

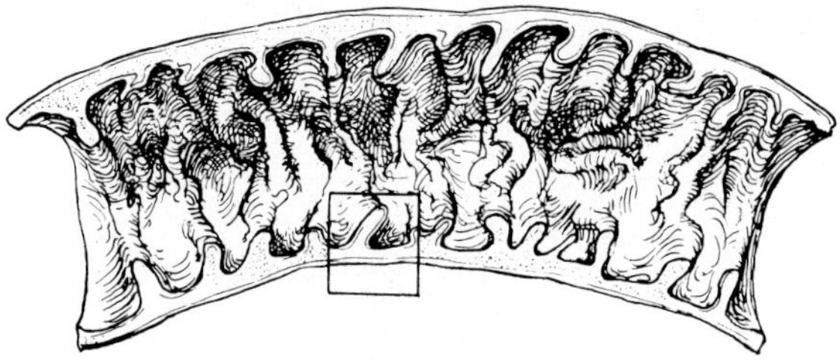

Figure 1–11. Macroscopical view of the inner aspect of the small intestine, showing the folds or valves of Kerckring. Each boxed-in area of Figures 1–11 through 1–13 is shown in greater magnification in the succeeding figure. (From Laster, L., and Ingelfinger, F. J.: New England J. Med. *264:*1138, 1961.)

MUCOSAL HISTOLOGY OF THE SMALL INTESTINE

Since absorption is one of the two primary functions of the small intestine, an acquaintance with the morphology of the mucous membrane of the small bowel is of importance. Figures 1–11 through 1–14 depict successively larger magnifications of the mucosa, beginning with a fold of Kerckring and ending with the brush border of a columnar absorbing cell.[6] Note the tremendous increase in absorbing surface afforded by the folds of Kerckring, the villi, and the brush border. Thus, the villi project into the lumen from the undulating folds of the valves of Kerckring. Each villus is lined by columnar absorbing cells which have on their luminal surface further folds of the brush border. Between the villi are the crypts of Lieber-

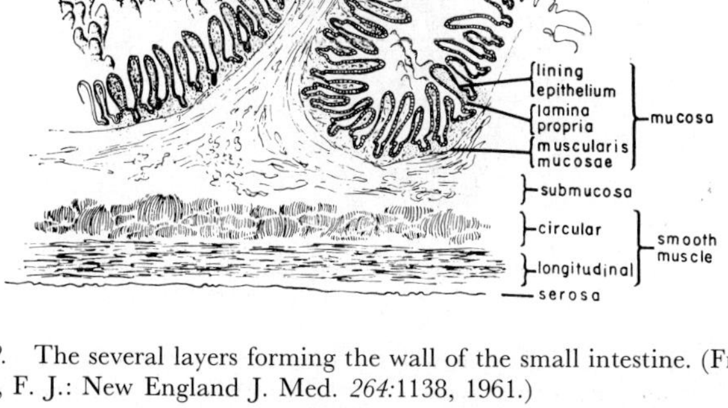

Figure 1–12. The several layers forming the wall of the small intestine. (From Laster, L., and Ingelfinger, F. J.: New England J. Med. *264:*1138, 1961.)

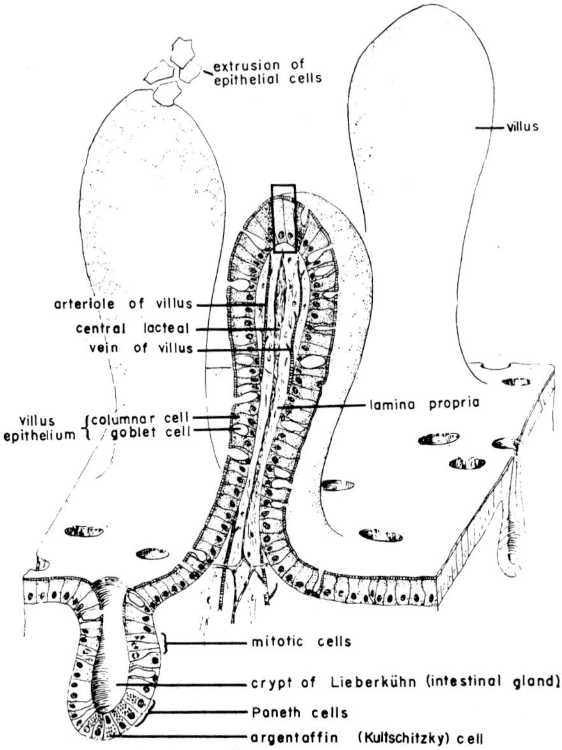

Figure 1–13. Three-dimensional reconstruction of the villi and the crypts of Lieberkühn. (From Laster, L., and Ingelfinger, F. J.: New England J. Med. *264:*1138, 1961.)

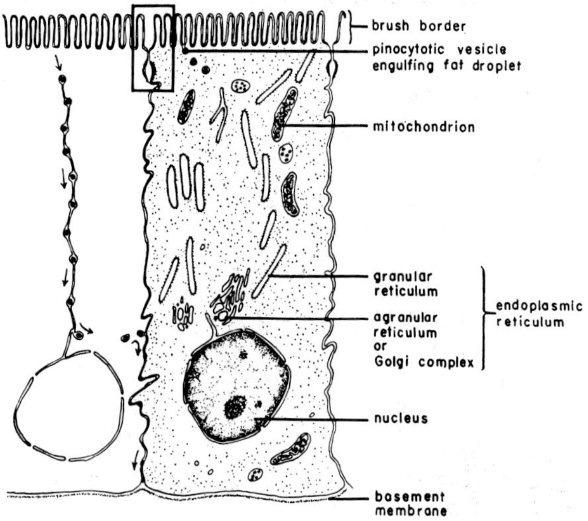

Figure 1–14. Highly schematic interpretation of the electron microscopic appearance of the columnar absorbing cell. (From Laster, L., and Ingelfinger, F. J.: New England J. Med. *264:*1139, 1961.)

kühn, thought to be the source of new columnar absorbing cells and goblet cells. In addition, they contain the Paneth's and argentaffin cells. Aside from a high concentration of serotonin in the latter[2] and other evidence for their being the probable precursor of carcinoid tumors of the small intestine, not much is known regarding these inhabitants of the crypts.

Histologically, the duodenum is unique in that Brunner's glands are prominent. Their terminal portions are made up of branched and coiled tubules which fuse into excretory ducts opening into the crypts of Lieberkühn.

Of prime importance in the villus are the central lacteal, the arteriole, and the venule. Absorbed substances find their way to these structures through the columnar cell for eventual delivery to the portal system or lymphatic trunk.

The presence of the intracellular particles, the mitochondria and the endoplasmic reticulum, has been defined and studied by means of electron microscopy. These bodies are concerned with absorption and with energy production in the formation of adenosine triphosphate.

REFERENCES

1. Alvarez, W. C.: An Introduction to Gastro-Enterology. Ed. 4. New York, Paul B. Hoeber, Inc., 1948.
2. Benditt, E. P., and Wong, R. L.: On concentration of 5-hydroxy-tryptamine in mammalian enterochromaffin cells and its release by reserpine. J. Exper. Med. *105:*509–520 (June 1) 1957.
3. Cattell, R. B., and Braasch, J. W.: A technique for the exposure of the third and fourth portions of the duodenum. Surg. Gynec. & Obst. *111:*378–379 (Sept.) 1960.
4. Gray, H.: Anatomy of the Human Body. Ed. 24. Edited by W. H. Lewis. Philadelphia, Lea & Febiger, 1942.
5. Hollinshead, W. H.: Anatomy for Surgeons. Vol. 2: The Thorax, Abdomen and Pelvis. New York, Paul B. Hoeber, Inc., 1956.
6. Laster, L., and Ingelfinger, F. J.: Intestinal absorption—aspects of structure, function and disease of the small-intestine mucosa. New England J. Med. *264:*1138–1148 (June 1) 1961.
7. Treves, F.: Lectures on the anatomy of the intestinal canal and peritoneum in man. Lectures I, II, and III. Brit. M. J. *1:*415–419, 470–474, 527–530 (Mar.) 1885.

Chapter Two

PHYSIOLOGY

The function of the small intestine is primarily nutritional. To this end it aids in the breakdown of more complex molecules to those simpler forms which it absorbs into the lymph or portal blood. These vital functions are accomplished by the production of enzymes important to this breakdown process, by providing a closed space that mixes the meal and renews and evacuates the luminal contents, and by providing an incredibly complex and efficient surface for absorption of a wide variety of compounds usable in the body economy. All these functions can be influenced by controls inside or outside of the bowel and are best discussed under the several headings of Mixing and Propulsion, Digestion, Absorption, Other Influences, and Localization of Absorption.

MIXING AND PROPULSION

Types of Contractions

The movements of the small intestine are provided for by two layers of smooth muscle in its wall, one longitudinal and one circular in orientation. The latter group is of primary importance. These muscles act in a remarkably rhythmic fashion so as to show two patterns of contraction. The first is described as being segmenting or pendular and serves to mix the contents of the bowel. The second is defined as peristalsis, the propulsive force of the small bowel. Usually the latter manifests itself by a progressive increase in tonus of the muscle without alteration in the segmenting and pendular movements. Occasionally, after exceedingly strong stimuli, a single peristaltic wave may sweep the entire length of the small intestine, or several such waves may occur in succession.

A third type of movement of the small intestine is that brought about by the muscularis mucosae that causes lashing, shortening, and lengthening movements of the intestinal villi. These movements are thought to be important for efficient absorption.

NATURAL FREQUENCY OF CONTRACTIONS

The "natural" frequency of the segmenting movements is lessened as the small intestine is descended. This frequency is surprisingly constant for any one area and is not markedly affected by stimulation of the extrinsic nerves or by neurotrophic drugs. Both mechanical and chemical stimuli are effective in promoting peristalsis and segmenting activity.

The mechanism underlying the rhythmicity and progression distally of intestinal contractions has intrigued physiologists for decades. Bayliss and Starling[5] described a "law of the intestine" to explain the small bowel peristaltic movements. Somewhat later Alvarez[2] proposed a "gradient theory" based on an inherent polarity of the intestine. In more recent times the explanations have become more sophisticated. Daniel et al.[15] and Hasselbrack and Thomas[26] have studied the electrical activity of the small bowel and described a duodenal pacemaker that exercises a measure of control.

ILEOCECAL VALVE

The ileocolic junction has two functions and two structures that expedite these functions. The passage of the chyme from the ileum into the cecum is delayed by the contraction and relaxation of the circular muscle fibers of the terminal ileum which are thickened in this area. This delay in evacuation of the small bowel enhances digestion and absorption.[21, 43] A second feature of the ileocecal junction is a mechanical valvelike device that permits flow from ileum into colon but, when competent, prevents cecal regurgitation into the ileum. This one-way valvelike action is accomplished by two transverse folds or lips, one above and the other below the cecal aspect of the ileocolic orifice. As the cecum distends, the lips are lengthened and drawn firmly together.

DIGESTION

GASTRIC AND PANCREATIC ENZYMES

It is in the small intestine that the breakdown of the large food components is completed to the forms of protein, carbohydrate, and fat that are most readily absorbed. Thus, as the chyme leaves the stomach, starch digestion is incomplete, fat digestion has barely begun, and the proteins are mostly in the form of large molecules containing many amino acids. The pancreatic enzymes include a potent lipase which probably renders fat fit for the absorption process; but pancreatic chymotrypsin, trypsin, and amylase leave proteins and sugars in the nonabsorbable forms, peptides and maltose.

SMALL INTESTINAL MUCOSAL ENZYMES

Enzymes whose source is the small intestinal mucosa complete the breakdown of peptides to amino acids and of various disaccharides to monosaccharides, which are easily absorbable. These enzymes include peptidases, lipases, and disaccharidases. The exact source of these enzymes is not known although most believe that they are primarily intracellular (columnar absorbing cell) originally and appear in the succus entericus after the disintegration and renewal of the columnar cells of the villus. Leblond and Walker[35] have pointed out that there is a continual turnover of the cells lining the villus, the renewal time being about two days. Thus in man, this breakdown and renewal has been calculated to contribute 250 gm. of tissue per day to the intestinal contents.

CRYPTS OF LIEBERKÜHN

The cells of the crypts of Lieberkühn have been shown to be the source of renewal of the columnar absorbing cells and the goblet cells of the villus. By certain histochemical techniques, the cells of the crypts can be shown to gain maturity as they approach the base of the villus.[50] The function of the Paneth cells of the crypt are unknown and little more is understood concerning the argentaffin cells. It has been demonstrated that the latter secrete serotonin or its precursor, 5-hydroxytryptophane, but the precise function of this compound is not known.

DUODENAL FUNCTIONS

The duodenal mucous membrane is unique in the small intestine as it contains in its proximal segments special mucous glands called Brunner's glands whose ducts empty into the crypts of Lieberkühn and secrete a lubricating mucus. Presumably their function is related to lubrication of the chyme and protection of the duodenal mucosa from acid peptic digestion.

The duodenum has other functions that make it unique in the small intestine. Its cells are thought to secrete an enzyme, enterokinase, which activates pancreatic trypsinogen in the duodenum.

Perhaps of more importance are the gastrointestinal tract hormones thought to originate from the duodenum. The first, secretin, discovered by Bayliss and Starling,[5] triggers a secretion of water and bicarbonates from the pancreas. Another substance that has been extracted from duodenal mucosa, pancreozymin, calls forth from the pancreas a secretion rich in enzymes. Stimuli for the elaboration of these hormones are afforded by hydrochloric acid, soaps, peptones, and even distilled water. Through these hormones the duodenal mucosa exercises a major controlling influence on pancreatic exocrine secretion. Other hormones extractable from the duodenal mucosa include cholecystokinin, which causes contraction of the gallbladder. Its formation is stimulated by the introduction of bile into the duodenum. The existence of a hormone stimulating bile secretion by the liver is not certain. The inhibiting effect on gastric secretion of low pH or fat in the duodenum is recognized. A hormone from the duodenum known as enterogastrone has been implicated in mediating the inhibition of gastric acid secretion in these circumstances.

The regulation of intestinal exogenous secretion is a controversial subject that includes the nervous and hormonal control of Brunner's gland secretion, enzyme secretion, and enterocrinin production. A full discussion of this subject is beyond the scope of this monograph.

ABSORPTION

Intestinal absorption is the complex process of transfer of the products of digestion into the lymphatic and portal systems. This area of physiology has received increasing attention in late years as specific deficits in absorption are recognized. For those surgeons dealing with small bowel insufficiency, it is of primary importance.

General Mechanisms

The student of the absorptive processes should refer to a monograph on "Intestinal Absorption" by Wilson[50] or to the articles by Laster and Ingelfinger[34] on the same subject. In general, there are believed to be four underlying mechanisms of translocation through the intestinal mucous membrane. These are passive diffusion, active transport, facilitated transport, and pinocytosis. Passive diffusion is that process responsible for the passage of a molecule across a membrane from a region of high concentration to one of low concentration. This process requires no expenditure of energy and is modified most importantly by the properties of the membrane crossed. It has been found that molecules that are highly lipid soluble can cross the intestinal membrane with much more efficiency than those with low solu-

Table 2–1. Comparison of Transport Capacity for Different Nutrients*

SUBSTANCE	ABSORPTIVE CAPACITY IN MAN PER DAY GRAMS	mM.
Water	18,000	1,000,000
Glucose	3,600	20,000
Amino acids	600	5,000
Triglycerides	700	900
Cholesterol	4	10
Iron	0.012	0.2
Vitamin B_{12}	0.000001	0.000001

* From Wilson, T. H.: Intestinal Absorption. Philadelphia, W. B. Saunders Co., 1962, p. 10.

bilities. There is disagreement as to the mechanism of absorption of water, some evidence supporting the concept that water moves by passive absorption and other evidence indicating the contrary.[34]

Active transport of a substance across the intestinal mucosa requires the cell to expend metabolic energy and implies the ability of a molecule to move against a concentration gradient. As a model of such absorption, one theory holds that the membrane to be traversed contains a carrier having chemical and spatial specificity that can pick up a substance on one side of the membrane and release it, chemically unchanged, on the opposite side. These processes require energy, which is most likely furnished by the adenosine triphosphate system of the cell.

The third variety, facilitated transport, resembles passive diffusion in that net movement occurs with gradients but, in addition, the degree of transport often exceeds that predictable from physical parameters.

Pinocytosis is that primitive mechanism for ingestion by engulfing particles or dissolved materials by vesiculation and thus is analagous to phagocytosis. There is some evidence that it is the method of absorption of triglycerides.[38]

As a model system, it is possible that transport across the mucosa of the small intestine might involve the following steps: binding of the substance to be absorbed to the surface of the columnar cell; transport across the apical surface of the membrane; intracellular metabolism and transcellular transport; release from the cell and migration across the basement membrane and the lamina propria with penetration of the portal venules or lacteals.[34] This multiplicity of processes involved might lead one to expect major differences in the absorptive capacity for differing compounds (Table 2–1).

MECHANISMS FOR SPECIFIC SUBSTANCES

Sugars are absorbed almost exclusively in the form of monosaccharides. Glucose and galactose are absorbed rapidly and can move against a concentration gradient. They are therefore thought to be absorbed by active transport.[40] Other compounds, such as mannose, sorbose, and pentose, are absorbed slowly and will not move against a gradient in the manner of passive absorption. Earlier work implicated phosphorylation as essential for absorption; however, there has never been conclusive proof of this concept. Disaccharides ordinarily cannot be absorbed intact and instead are split into their respective monosaccharides, probably by the cells of the mucous membrane and not the succus entericus.[14]

Our knowledge of lipid absorption is far from complete.[34] The evidence for and against a particular mechanism is voluminous. In addition, the lipids are a heterogeneous group of compounds and apparently are absorbed by differing mechanisms. A review of the pertinent literature is given by Laster and Ingelfinger[34] and Dawson and Isselbacher.[16] The latter authors believe that after an extensive but incomplete hydrolysis of neutral fat in the lumen of the small intestine by pancreatic lipase and bile salts, 70 percent of the fatty acid is liberated and subsequently absorbed in the free form. Thirty percent of the fatty acid passes into the mucosal cell as glycerides. Pinocytosis or phagocytosis of the lipid droplet by the columnar cell accounts for part of the lipid mixture absorbed by the cell. The short chain fatty acids pass from the columnar cell into the portal blood, and the long chain fatty acids are esterified with glycerol and incorporated into chylomicrons which are discharged into the lymphatics. Bile salts, adenosine triphosphate, coenzyme A, and magnesium ions are important in membrane passage and intracellar metabolism in the intestinal mucosa.

In perspective, fatty acids with short carbon chains tend to be more efficiently absorbed or utilized than those with longer carbon chains. Unsaturated fatty acids enjoy a like advantage over the saturated chains.

As for other lipids, phospholipids are absorbed largely via the lymphatics, up to 25 percent in the intact form. Cholesterol is likewise efficiently absorbed by the small intestine via the lymphatics. The presence of bile salts is necessary for this absorption.

Proteins are almost completely absorbed as amino acids. In general the l-isomers are more rapidly absorbed and can move against a concentration gradient.[51] Lack of vitamin B seems to retard amino acid absorption, a deficiency correctable by pyridoxine administration.[30] The intestinal mucosa is the site of an intense protein synthesis, the exact relationship of which to the absorption process is unknown. The end pathway of amino acid absorption is the portal vein.

The exact mechanism of the amino acid pump or transport mechanism is unknown, but from studies on patients with genetic defects, it appears that there are several varying pathways for basic amino acids, neutral amino acids, proline and hydroxyproline, and perhaps glycine.[12]

The work of Visscher et al.[47] demonstrated the fact that there is a bidirectional flow of water and electrolytes between the blood and gut. The magnitude of these rates was further explored by Scholer and Code[42] and Code et al.,[11] who estimated the rate of insorption of water to be 20 percent of the ingested amount per minute in the animal and human small intestine. The corresponding rate for sodium is approximately 10 percent. The evidence for and against the active or passive insorption of water is controversial. It is probable that both methods are available. There is fair agreement, however, that electrolyte transport is an active process, perhaps associated with mitochondria binding.[47] Water and electrolytes are absorbed almost entirely into the portal blood.

The rate of intestinal absorption of divalent cations such as calcium is much slower than that for sodium or chloride. Vitamin D is essential for calcium absorption with normal or low calcium intakes.[41] Transport across the gut wall can be accomplished against a gradient requiring oxidative phosphorylation in addition to vitamin D. It is surmised that parahormone plays an important part in this transfer.

Iron absorption is unique in that its assimilation is dependent on the organism's needs.[37] It is obligatory that the commonly found ferric form be reduced to ferrous iron before absorption can take place. The most effective reducing agent in the gastrointestinal tract is hydrochloric acid; however, bile can also reduce iron from its ferric state to the ferrous form. The ferrous ion then enters the mucosal cell where it is oxidized to ferric iron and where it combines with the protein, apoferritin. Combination with this protein is essential for absorption, and when the limited supply of apoferritin is filled, no more absorption of iron can take place. Iron traverses the cell in combination with ferritin and is released from this combination into the portal blood.

The water soluble vitamins, nicotinamide, pyridoxine, inositol, ascorbic acid, choline, para-aminobenzoic acid, biotin, pantothenic acid, riboflavin, thiamine, and folic acid, probably pass across the intestinal wall by simple diffusion. In general, the smaller the molecule (such as inositol, biotin, and ascorbic acid) the greater is the absorptive capacity of the intestine. Those molecules with strong ionization (thiamine) are poorly absorbed.

Vitamin B_{12} is absorbed in three phases. First, the vitamin is bound to intrinsic factor which is found in the gastric juice. The second phase involves the attachment of the intrinsic factor–vitamin B_{12} complex to the intestinal mucosa, a process greatly enhanced by the presence of calcium ions.[27, 28] Third, there is the transport of absorbed vitamin B_{12} across the mucosa and into the portal blood. In vivo studies have indicated that there is up to a four hour delay during which the vitamin remains within the intestinal wall.[19]

The fat soluble vitamins, A, D, K, and E, are probably absorbed by mechanisms similar to those for lipid absorption. Thus, bile salts are essential for adequate absorption, indicating that emulsification is important. There is no evidence for any specialized transport mechanism, and it seems likely that absorption takes place by diffusion. An important source for vitamin K is the bacterial flora of the intestine. Thus alteration of this flora by the

Table 2-2. Comparative Importance of Active Transport and Passive Diffusion in Intestinal Absorption*

SUBSTANCE	FRACTION ABSORBED BY ACTIVE TRANSPORT
NaCl (and H_2O)	Very large
Glucose	Large
Amino acids	Large
Fats	Large
Vitamins	Little or none (except B_{12})
Nucleic acid derivatives	Little (except uracil and thymine)

* Adapted from Wilson, T. H.: Intestinal Absorption. Philadelphia, W. B. Saunders Co., 1962, p. 51.

administration of antibiotics may produce deficiencies of this vitamin. It is interesting that carotene can be substituted for vitamin A in the diet. It seems likely that the intestinal mucosal columnar cell can convert carotene into vitamin A.[36]

A summary of the transport mechanism for most substances is found in Table 2-2.

OTHER INFLUENCES ON FUNCTION

The influence of nervous impulses on the small intestine has many implications for clinical surgery. Earlier studies on the effects of vagotomy in animals have been summarized by Alvarez[3] (1948), who found a complete lack of agreement in this area. Most early authors were interested in the effect on intestinal motility as were Faik et al.,[20] who noted that the activity of the dog's intestine occurring at the sight and smell of food was absent after vagotomy. In addition, the peristaltic waves were fewer, of shorter duration, and occurred at longer intervals. Ballinger et al.[4] have noted atrophy of the mucosa of the small intestine with reduction in the mucosal enzyme concentration in dogs following bilateral abdominal vagotomy. These changes were maximal three weeks postoperatively, but were reversible, and recovery was complete 12 to 21 weeks after operation. In further studies in dogs, Tucker et al.[46] compared fat, protein, and carbohydrate absorption after pyloroplasty with and without various types of vagotomy. They noted little influence of the vagotomy.

The clinical response of patients with regional enteritis and ulcerative colitis following vagotomy was observed by Dennis et al.[18] In the opinion of these authors there was a favorable response to this operation as judged by well-being and number of bowel movements. Longer follow-up has not borne this out. After vagotomy in humans, Issac et al.[29] found dilatation of the duodenum, jejunum, and ileum, and segmentation, pooling, and flocculation of barium with delay in intestinal motility. In the opinion of Wollaeger et al.,[52] vagotomy alone does not produce steatorrhea but it might make manifest a latent tendency due to other causes.

It seems likely, therefore, that there is little permanent change in small intestinal function after vagotomy, although there is some sentiment to the contrary.[25, 45] The histologic and anatomic changes seem to be reversible.

Various other influences on the absorptive process have been assessed. These include blood flow to the intestine,[9, 23] the concentration of villi in a given length of intestine (there are fewer in the ileum),[16] the effect of gastric hypersecretion in causing steatorrhea,[39] the effect of the pH in the upper small bowel (acid pH decreases glucose absorption),[22] the effect of the ileocecal valve in promoting absorption,[32] the effect of hypermotility,[32, 44] the effect of more thorough mixing in the upper small intestine,[13] and the control on absorption exerted by hormones or nervous influences.

LOCALIZATION OF ABSORPTION

The exact localization of the various absorptive functions of the small intestine has received increased attention from both the laboratory and the clinical standpoint. In planning and following sidetracking or resective procedures this information has obvious importance. Our knowledge of the sites of absorption is fragmentary in some areas and controversial in others. It is obtained from observations on patients who have had various portions of the small intestine resected or defunctionalized; from normal subjects in whom several "pure" substances have been introduced into the bowel at various levels and the intestinal contents sampled at lower levels; from balance studies in patients and animals; and from in vitro studies using homogenates of intestinal mucosa or everted lengths of animal intestine.

Carbohydrate, Fat, and Protein

It would seem from a careful review of the available information that in man the entire small intestine is capable of absorbing carbohydrate, fat, and protein. Ordinarily, however, the ileum fulfills this function only in the presence of high intakes or following resection of the jejunum.[6, 7, 8, 10, 13] This generalization holds true for test meals of corn oil, glucose, and milk proteins;[8] but in the digestion and absorption of complex mixtures dealt with in an ordinary meal, the proper digestion for absorption may not have occurred for some components until the ileum is reached. The disaccharides were studied by Dahlqvist and Borgström[14] in man, using intestinal tubes to administer and sample, and their results are somewhat at variance with the foregoing. They pointed out that the disaccharides are hydrolyzed by the cells of the intestinal mucous membrane and the monosaccharides formed within the cell are secreted into the portal vein. They plotted the sites of absorption as follows: for lactose—duodenum and proximal jejunum, for maltose—jejunum and proximal ileum, and for sucrose—distal jejunum and ileum. In a clinical study by Kalser et al.[32] of patients who had resection of various lengths and portions of the small intestine, the opposite conclusion was reached—that the ileum was the primary site of absorption of fat and nitrogen.

In general, animal studies involving dogs and rats confirm the majority of the human studies in that the upper small intestine is the major fat, carbohydrate, and protein absorber in the normal subject, but that the ileum is capable of absorbing these substances also.[7, 24, 31] Conversely, Kremen et al.,[33] working with dogs, found that the distal small intestine was of more importance in fat absorption after a 50 percent mesenteric small bowel resection.

The prevailing opinion as to the preferential site for absorption of fat in the jejunum, is borne out by studies showing that cell-free homogenates of rat and human intestinal mucosa from the duodenum or jejunum were four or five times as active in this regard as those from the ileum.[17]

VITAMIN B_{12} AND BILE SALTS

The ileum has been demonstrated in man[1] and in the rat[27, 28] to be the principal site of vitamin B_{12} absorption. The specificity of this portion of the small intestine in this function is unique, as the duodenum and jejunum appear to be incapable of absorbing this compound. The ileum also shows a unique absorption capability for bile salts.[48]

IRON

The importance of the upper small bowel in iron absorption has been demonstrated.[37] Apparently this feature of the upper bowel is dependent on its acid pH, because when the ileum is transposed with the duodenum and jejunum, it also shows this property.[49]

Table 2–3, adapted from Wilson,[50] and Figure 2–1 summarize our knowledge of the localization of specific compound absorption. It is to be noted that except for vitamin B_{12} and the bile salts, which are almost exclusively absorbed in the ileum, in the normal subject most of the absorption of fat, carbohydrate, protein, vitamins, and iron is carried out in the upper small intestine.

Table 2–3. Active Transport of Substances by the Intestine and Location of Maximum Absorption*

Substance	Location of absorptive capacity Small intestine *Upper*	 *Middle*	 *Lower*
Sugars	+ +	+ + +	+ +
Amino acids	+ + +	+ + +	+ +
Triglycerides	+ +	+ +	+
Fatty acid with conversion to triglycerides	+ + +	+ +	+
Betaine, dimethylglycine, sarcosine	+ +	+ +	+ +
Pyrimidines	+	+	?
Bile salts	0	+	+ + +
Vitamin B_{12}	0	+	+ + +
Na^+	+ + +	+ +	+ + +
H^+	0	+	+ +
Ca^{++}	+ + +	+ +	+
Fe^{++}	+ + +	+ +	+
Cl^-	+ + +	+ +	+
SO_4^{--}	+ +	+	0

*Adapted from Wilson, T. H.: Intestinal Absorption. Philadelphia, W. B. Saunders Co., 1962, p. 52.

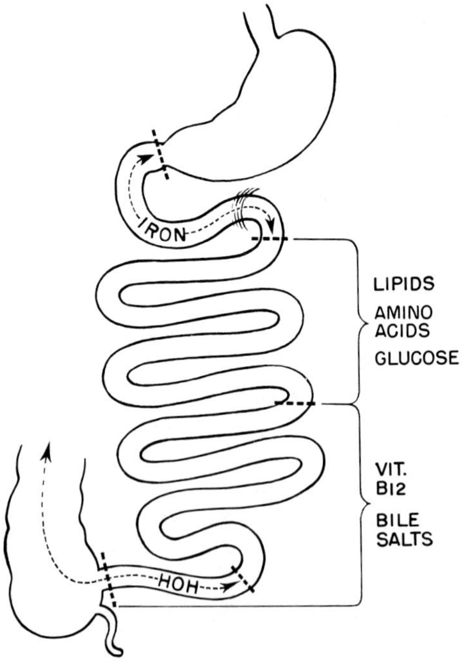

Figure 2–1. Sites of absorption of various substances.

REFERENCES

1. Allcock, E.: Absorption of vitamin B_{12} in man following extensive resection of the jejunum and colon. Gastroenterology *40:*81–85 (Jan.) 1961.
2. Alvarez, W. C.: The metabolic gradient underlying peristalsis. J.A.M.A. *73:*1438–1440 (Nov. 8) 1919.
3. Alvarez, W. C.: Sixty years of vagotomy; review of some 200 articles. Gastroenterology *10:*413–441 (Mar.) 1948.
4. Ballinger, W. F., II, Iida, J., Aponte, G. E., et al.: Structure and function of the canine small intestine following total abdominal vagotomy. Surg. Gynec. & Obst. *118:*1305–1311 (June) 1964.
5. Bayliss, W. M., and Starling, E. H.: The movements and innervation of the small intestine. J. Physiol. *24:*99–143 (May 11) 1899.
6. Booth, C. C., Alldis, D., and Read, A. E.: Studies on the site of fat absorption. 2. Fat balances after resection of varying amounts of the small intestine in man. Gut *2:*168–174 (June) 1961.
7. Booth, C. C., Read, A. E., and Jones, E.: Studies on the site of fat absorption. 1. The sites of absorption of increasing doses of 131-I-labelled triolein in the rat. Gut *2:*23–31 (Mar.) 1961.
8. Borgström, B., Dahlqvist, A., Lundh, G., and Sjovall, J.: Studies of intestinal digestion and absorption in the human. J. Clin. Invest. *36:*1521–1536 (Oct.) 1957.
9. Brandt, J. L., et al.: Effect of oral protein and glucose feeding on splanchnic blood flow and oxygen utilization in normal and cirrhotic subjects. J. Clin. Invest. *34:*1017–1025 (July) pt. 1 1955.
10. Brooks, F. P.: Absorption of protein, fat, and carbohydrate and their digestion products from the small intestine. Am. J. Gastroenterol. *36:*133–142 (Aug.) 1961.
11. Code, C. F., Bass, P., McClary, G. B., Jr., Newnum, R. L., and Orvis, A. L.: Absorption of water, sodium and potassium in small intestine of dogs. Am. J. Physiol. *199:*281–288 (Aug.) 1960.
12. Cooper, B. A., and Castle, W. B.: Sequential mechanisms in the enhanced absorption of vitamin B_{12} by intrinsic factor in the rat. J. Clin. Invest. *39:*199–214 (Jan.) 1960.
13. Cummins, A. J., and Jussila, R.: Comparison of glucose absorption rates in upper and lower human small intestine. Gastroenterology *29:*982–992 (Dec.) 1955.
14. Dahlqvist, A., and Borgström, B.: Digestion and absorption of disaccharides in man. Biochem. J. *81:*411–418 (Nov.) 1961.
15. Daniel, E. E., Carlow, D. R., Wachter, B. T., Sutherland, W. H., and Bogoch, A.: Electrical activity of the small intestine. Gastroenterology *37:*268–281 (Sept.) 1959.
16. Dawson, A. M., and Isselbacher, K. J.: The esterification of palmitate I-C14 by homogenates of intestinal mucosa. J. Clin. Invest. *39:*150–160 (Jan.) 1960.
17. Dawson, A. M., and Isselbacher, K. J.: Fat absorption. Arch. Int. Med. *107:*305–308 (Feb.) 1961.
18. Dennis, C., et al.: Response to vagotomy in idiopathic ulcerative colitis and regional enteritis. Ann. Surg. *128:*479–496 (Sept.) 1948.
19. Doscherholmen, A., and Hagen, P. S.: A dual mechanism of vitamin B_{12} plasma absorption. J. Clin. Invest. *36:*1551–1557 (Oct.) 1957.
20. Faik, S., Grindlay, J. H., and Mann, F. C.: Effect of vagotomy on intestinal activity. Surgery *28:*546–549 (Sept.) 1950.
21. Gazet, J. C., and Koop, J.: The surgical significance of the ileocecal junction. Surgery *56:*565–573 (Sept.) 1964.
22. Goldenberg, J., and Cummins, A. J.: The effect of pH on the absorption rate of glucose in the small intestine of humans. Gastroenterology *45:*189–195 (Aug.) 1963.
23. Groisser, V. W., and Farrar, J. T.: Absorption of radioactive sodium from the intestinal tract of man. I. Effect of intestinal motility. II. Effect of an organomercurial. J. Clin. Invest. *39:*1607–1618 (Nov.) 1960.
24. Gump, F., Beals, R., and Barker, H. G.: Effect of small intestinal resection on fat absorption. Ann. Surg. *154:*417–423 (Sept.) 1961.
25. Harkins, H. N., Stavney, L. S., Griffith, C. A., et al.: Selective gastric vagotomy. Ann. Surg. *158:*448–460 (Sept.) 1963.

26. Hasselbrack, R., and Thomas, J. E.: Control of intestinal rhythmic contractions by a duodenal pacemaker. Am. J. Physiol. *201:*955–960 (Nov.) 1961.
27. Herbert, V.: Mechanism of intrinsic factor action in everted sacs of rat small intestine. J. Clin. Invest. *38:*102–109 (Jan.) 1959.
28. Herbert, V., Cooper, B. A., and Castle, W. B.: The site of vitamin B_{12}–intrinsic factor complex "releasing factor" activity in the rat small intestine. Proc. Soc. Exper. Biol. & Med. *110:*315–317 (June) 1962.
29. Issac, F., Ottoman, R. E., and Weinberg, J. A.: Roentgen studies of upper gastrointestinal tract in vagotomy. Am. J. Roentgenol. *63:*66–75 (Jan.) 1950.
30. Jacobs, F. A., Coen, L. J., and Hillman, R. S.: Influence of pyridoxine, pyridoxal phosphate, deoxypyridoxine and 2,4-dinitrophenol on methionine absorption. J. Biol. Chem. *235:*1372–1375 (May) 1960.
31. Johnston, J. M.: Site of fatty acid absorption. Proc. Soc. Exper. Biol. & Med. *100:*669–670 (Apr.) 1959.
32. Kalser, M. H., Roth, J. L., Tumen, H., and Johnson, T. A.: Relation of small bowel resection to nutrition in man. Gastroenterology *38:*605–615 (Apr.) 1960.
33. Kremen, A. J., Linner, J. H., and Nelson, C. H.: An experimental evaluation of nutritional importance of proximal and distal small intestine. Ann. Surg. *140:*439–448 (Sept.) 1954.
34. Laster, L., and Ingelfinger, F. J.: Intestinal absorption–aspects of structure, function and disease of the small-intestine mucosa. New England J. Med. *264:*1138–1148 (June 1); 1192–1200 (June 8) 1961.
35. Leblond, C. P., and Walker, B. E.: Renewal of cell populations. Physiol. Rev. *36:*255–276 (Apr.) 1956.
36. Lowe, J. S., and Morton, R. A.: Some aspects of vitamin A metabolism. Vitamins & Hormones *14:*97–137, 1956.
37. Noyes, W. D., and Jordan, P. H.: Small bowel iron absorption in an unusual patient. Gastroenterology *46:*421–423 (Apr.) 1964.
38. Palay, S. L., and Karlin, L. J.: An electron microscopic study of the intestinal villus. II. The pathway of fat absorption. J. Biophys. Cytol. *5:*373–384 (May 25) 1959.
39. Preshaw, R. M., and Fisher, A. G.: Steatorrhea in dogs induced by gastric hypersecretion. Surg. Gynec. & Obst. *118:*31–37 (Jan.) 1964.
40. Quastel, J. H.: Intestinal absorption of sugars and amino acids. Am. J. Clin. Nutrition *8:*137–146 (Mar.-Apr.) 1960.
41. Schachter, D., and Rosen, S. M.: Active transport of Ca^{45} by the small intestine and its dependence on vitamin D. Am. J. Physiol. *196:*357–362 (Feb.) 1959.
42. Scholer, J. F., and Code, C. F.: Rate of absorption of water from stomach and small bowel of human beings. Gastroenterology *27:*565–577 (Nov.) 1954.
43. Singleton, A. O., Jr., Redmond, D. C., II, and McMurray, J. E.: Ileocecal resection and small bowel transit and absorption. Ann. Surg. *159:*690–694 (May) 1964.
44. Stahlgren, L. H., Umana, G., Roy, R., and Donnelly, J.: A study of intestinal absorption in dogs following massive small intestinal resection and insertion of an antiperistaltic segment. Ann. Surg. *156:*483–492 (Sept.) 1962.
45. Stavney, L. S., Kato, T., Griffith, C. A., et al.: A physiologic study of motility changes following selective gastric vagotomy. J. Surg. Research *3:*390–394 (Oct.) 1963.
46. Tucker, F. H., Barnett, W. O., and Goodrich, J.: The influence of various degrees of vagotomy upon fat, carbohydrate, and protein absorption following pyloroplasty. Surg. Gynec. & Obst. *118:*1281–1285 (June) 1964.
47. Visscher, M. B., Fetcher, E. S., Jr., Carr, C. W., Gregor, H. P., Bushey, M. S., and Barker, D. E.: Isotopic tracer studies on movement of water and ions between intestinal lumen and blood. Am. J. Physiol. *142:*550–575 (Nov.) 1944.
48. Weiner, I. M., and Lack, L.: Absorption of bile salts from the small intestine in vivo. Am. J. Physiol. *202:*155–157 (Jan.) 1962.
49. Williams, J. S., Spencer, R., and Drapanas, T.: Effect of duodenal and jejunal transposition on iron absorption in the dog. S. Forum *14:*370–371, 1963.
50. Wilson, T. H.: Intestinal Absorption. Philadelphia, W. B. Saunders Co., 1962, 263 pp.
51. Wiseman, G.: Absorption of amino-acids using in vitro technique. J. Physiol. *120:*63–72 (Apr.) 1953.
52. Wollaeger, E. E., Waugh, J. M., and Power, M. H.: Fat-assimilating capacity of the gastrointestinal tract after partial gastrectomy with gastroduodenostomy (Billroth I anastomosis). Gastroenterology *44:*25–32 (Jan.) 1963.

Chapter Three

OBSTRUCTION

GENERAL ASPECTS AND CLASSIFICATION

Obstruction of the small intestine can be and often is a catastrophic event. The use of the long gastrointestinal tube for decompression of the bowel has undoubtedly saved lives and represents a great advance; but its improper use has resulted in many deaths. The lack of appreciation by the attending physician of the potential hazard inherent in small bowel obstruction often leads to delay in treatment, and delay in treatment in certain instances is fatal. Nine thousand deaths due to small intestinal obstruction are recorded yearly in this country.[102] Sequential studies of the results of treatment of small bowel obstruction have shown that the mortality rate has not declined in the last 15 years and approximates 15 percent. Certainly, the serious problem of small bowel obstruction is still with us.

The classification of acute obstruction of the small intestine is of great importance as an aid in both the understanding of this subject and the practical management of a case of obstruction (Table 3–1). Of the various causes of obstruction outlined, the most common are adhesions or bands, followed by hernias. The merging of chronic with acute obstruction and the overlay of factors characteristic of each, preclude an orderly discussion of each of these types of obstruction. Therefore, the area of acute obstruction will receive the most attention in this chapter. It should be recognized that the difference between the two types is simply one of degree.

The usual division of cases is into those spoken of as dynamic or mechanical obstruction and the variety known variously as ileus, adynamic ileus, or paralytic ileus. In the former situation a lesion produces actual occlusion of the intestinal lumen and prevents the orderly progression of fluids and gases through the intestine. In the latter situation, the clinical management is vastly different from that in the former. Thus, it is

Table 3–1. Causes of Acute Small Intestinal Obstruction*

- I. Mechanical Occlusion of Lumen
  - A. Intrinsic defects of intestine
    - 1. Congenital defects
      - a. Errors in rotation of intestine
      - b. Duplications and cysts
      - c. Meckel's diverticulum
    - 2. Inflammatory lesions
      - a. Regional enteritis
      - b. Tuberculosis
      - c. Diverticulitis
      - d. Eosiniphilic granuloma
    - 3. Tumors
      - a. Benign
      - b. Malignant
    - 4. Traumatic lesions
      - a. Strictures
      - b. Hematomas
    - 5. Intussusception
    - 6. Radiation strictures
    - 7. Endometriosis
    - 8. Pneumatosis intestinales
  - B. Obturation obstruction
    - 1. Gallstones
    - 2. Bezoars
    - 3. Foreign bodies
    - 4. Enteroliths
    - 5. Worms
    - 6. Balloons of intestinal tubes
  - C. Volvulus
    - 1. Primary
    - 2. Secondary
      - a. Associated congenital abnormality
      - b. Secondary surgical artifact
      - c. Secondary bands, adhesions, stenosis, or obturation
  - D. Extraintestinal lesions
    - 1. Adhesions and bands
    - 2. Hernia
      - a. Extraabdominal
        Inguinal, femoral, umbilical, ventral, diaphragmatic, lumbar, epigastric, interstitial, prevesical, obturator, sciatic, perineal, Richter's, Littre's
      - b. Intraabdominal
        Paraduodenal, foramen of Winslow, paracecal, intersigmoid, through omental or mesenteric defect, through broad ligament
    - 3. Compression by extraintestinal mass
      - a. Carcinomatosis
      - b. Intraperitoneal abscess
      - c. Adjacent tumor
      - d. Pregnancy
      - e. Foreign body
      - f. Superior mesenteric artery duodenal obstruction
      - g. Annular pancreas
      - h. Wandering spleen
  - E. Obstruction secondary to surgical operation (other than adhesions)
    - 1. Intraperitoneal abscess
    - 2. Wound dehiscence
    - 3. Anastomotic obstruction (stricture or edema)
    - 4. Anastomotic leak

Table 3–1. Causes of Acute Small Intestinal Obstruction* (*Continued*)

5. Obstruction at external stoma
6. Hernia through trap or peritoneal defect
7. Volvulus about fixed point

II. Obstruction With Open Lumen
   A. Paralytic ileus
   B. Spastic ileus
   C. Mesenteric vascular occlusion

*Adapted from Welch, C. E.: Intestinal Obstruction. Chicago, Year Book Medical Publishers, Inc., 1958, pp. 50–51. Used by permission of Year Book Medical Publishers, Inc.

enormously important for the clinician to decide: first, "is obstruction of the intestine present," and second, "is the case one of mechanical obstruction or so-called adynamic ileus." This decision can be most difficult in certain situations. Compounding the difficulty can be the fact that one type of obstruction can complicate the other.

Of further importance is the differentiation of strangulating from simple mechanical obstruction; the former demands emergency surgery, and the latter permits a more leisurely approach with time for correction of fluid deficits and attempts at long tube decompression.[13, 94]

PATHOLOGIC PHYSIOLOGY

GENERAL SEQUENCE OF EVENTS

The lack of normal progression of intestinal contents is the basis for intestinal obstruction. Several interrelated derangements in small bowel function and other areas of the internal milieu ensue.[13, 56] Of primary importance is the accumulation of intestinal contents proximal to the obstructed area. Normally the secretions of the upper gastrointestinal tract amount to about 8 liters of fluid a day.[41, 65] Since reabsorption of water is negligible in the stomach and upper small bowel and appreciable only throughout the distal small bowel and cecum, the continued delivery to the obstructed point of a large volume of fluid quickly causes dilatation of the intestine. This volume of fluid when added to accumulated intestinal gas from swallowed air can in a matter of hours produce marked distention of the bowel proximal to the obstruction.[48, 65, 108] Associated with distention is venous obstruction,[37] edema of the bowel wall, and according to some authorities, an increase in secretion of fluids into the affected loop.[30] The usual result if the obstruction is high in the small intestine is vomiting and loss of extracellular fluid, immediate and of marked degree. It is obvious that with lesser degrees of obstruction, these changes are of lesser magnitude and immediacy. Likewise, obstruction low in the ileum manifests itself less by immediate vomiting and more by abdominal distention. With increasing

Table 3–2. Source and Composition of Intestinal Fluids*

	24-HOUR OUTPUT	COMPOSITION (MEQ./L.)				
	(cc.)	*Na*	*Cl*	*K*	*HCO_3*	*Mg*
Saliva	1500	9	10	26	15	
Gastric juice	2500	25	150	12	0	1
Bile	500	140	100	10	30	
Pancreatic juice	700	140	75	10	75	
Succus entericus	3000	140	105	10	25	

*Adapted from Gamble, J. L.: Chemical Anatomy, Physiology and Pathology of Extracellular Fluids: A Lecture Syllabus. Ed. 6. Cambridge, Harvard University Press, 1954, pp. 115, 117.

distention there is also an increase in intraabdominal pressure. This results in elevation of the diaphragm and lowering of vital capacity. In addition, in extreme instances a reduction in venous return via the inferior vena cava and diminution of portal vein flow ensue.[12, 40]

FLUID AND ELECTROLYTE DISTURBANCES AND TREATMENT

Table 3–2 gives information on the amount, content and source of the various fluids found in the lumen of obstructed loops of small intestine.[41] It is apparent that high duodenal obstructions will be followed by loss of a fluid relatively rich in chloride, most of which is of gastric origin, whereas obstructions low in the small intestine feature electrolyte loss of a composition similar to extracellular fluid.[13, 56, 72] Therefore, replacement of upper small intestinal losses should consist in part of fluid containing appreciable concentrations of NH_4Cl. The ammonium ion is metabolized leaving the excess chloride for replacement of ionic chloride deficit. Replacement solutions for lower small intestine losses are generally similar to extracellular fluid. Attention should also be paid to potassium and occasionally magnesium replacement[59] especially in cases of chronic losses. The availability of concentrated salt solutions, 3 or 5 percent, for replacement of severe deficits should be recognized. Monographs on fluid and electrolyte metabolism should be consulted for more complex problems.[15, 76]

STRANGULATION OBSTRUCTION

As the intestinal gas and secretions accumulate within the lumen of the obstructed bowel, the rise in pressure within the bowel is accommodated by dilatation of the bowel wall.[13, 56] With or without a twist in the loop of involved bowel which prevents proximal dilatation, extensive disruption of the normal vascular supply can follow extensive dilatation, and anoxia of the bowel wall ensues. Perforation of the bowel is then possible, especially where the blood supply to the involved loop is compromised. Should this occur, death from peritonitis and shock is nearly inevitable.

There may be extensive blood, plasma, or extracellular fluid loss into the lumen or strangulated bowel wall. In the experimental animal, losses up to 48 percent of the plasma volume or 28 percent of the blood volume have been noted.[42]

Even without rupture of the bowel wall, the intraluminal contents can be in part absorbed into the general circulation. There is some difference of opinion as to just what the substance is which is so lethal to the organism upon its entry into the general circulation.[28, 78, 79, 99, 113] Porphyrin compounds, bacterial endotoxins, exotoxin, and the bacterial organisms themselves have all been implicated. It seems likely that there is a relationship between toxicity and bacterial growth within the strangulated loop since treatment with antibiotics abolishes this specific toxic effect, and studies of peritoneal fluid of dogs with strangulated obstruction indicate that the toxic factor is related to the bacterial content of the centrifugate. For a comprehensive review of this subject, the reader is referred to Cohn.[27]

MALABSORPTION

Since the first report in 1895 of a pernicious anemia-like syndrome occurring in a patient with intestinal stricture and chronic obstruction, other evidences of a malabsorption syndrome associated with chronic obstruction have been found.[39] Thus steatorrhea and a variety of hypovitaminosis states have been reported.[44, 61, 100] In addition to chronic obstruction, blind loops and diverticula are associated with malabsorption. The common denominator seems to be stasis of intestinal contents with a relationship to an overgrowth of intestinal flora. For a fuller discussion of this subject the reader is referred to the chapter on diverticula of the small intestine.

DIAGNOSIS OF OBSTRUCTION

FEATURES OF HIGH, LOW, AND STRANGULATING OBSTRUCTION

The symptoms, physical findings, and laboratory and radiologic findings of the patient with acute small intestinal obstruction are usually characteristic.[56] Intermittent cramping abdominal pain and nausea with or without vomiting are the hallmarks of acute intestinal obstruction. With partial obstruction, diarrhea may be prominent. More likely, there is cessation of bowel action and failure to pass gas rectally. The character of the vomitus may be light and watery with high small bowel obstruction, and dark and foul-smelling with low ileal lesions. The physical findings vary with the site and character of the obstruction. Thus, with high obstructions there is little if any distention, whereas with low obstructions distention is prominent. Usually, unless there is impairment of bowel wall viability, there is no or little abdominal tenderness; however, occasionally the discomfort of distention is increased by palpation. As a rule, definite tenderness and abdominal wall muscular spasm is elicitable only with strangulating obstructions.[13] Occasionally with strangulating obstruction an abdominal mass is palpable, representing a closed loop of questionable viability. Auscultation of the abdomen is usually clinically useful. Traditionally, high-pitched sounds are considered characteristic of mechanical obstruction and are frequently coincident with a cramping pain. The silent abdomen signifies peritonitis or "ileus" or "paralytic ileus."

RADIOLOGIC DIAGNOSIS

X-ray observations of the abdomen are of extreme importance in the diagnosis of obstruction, in locating the obstruction, and at times in defining the cause of obstruction. Radiographs should be obtained with the patient in the horizontal and, in addition, in either upright or lateral decubitus positions. Care must be taken that the diaphragm and the pelvis are included in the films. Traditionally, the presence of gas in the small bowel in increased amounts with dilatation of the small bowel and fluid levels therein on the upright films are pathognomonic of small bowel obstruction (Figs. 3–1, 3–2, and 3–3). At times, a mass may be visualized in the abdomen that is suggestive of a strangulated loop of bowel. Frequently, the thickness of the bowel wall can be appreciated on plain films of the abdomen, which can give insight into the degree and progress of the obstruction (Fig. 3–1). The differentiation on the plain horizontal radiograph of small from large bowel distention is of importance. Characteristically, the fine banding of the gas shadow extends from one side of the small bowel to the other (Fig. 3–1); whereas, in a dilated colon the bands are irregular and do not traverse the bowel shadow (Fig. 3–4).

The cause of obstruction can occasionally be discovered from inspection of the plain film of the abdomen. The hallmarks of gallstone ileus, air in the biliary tree with a concretion in the bowel lumen, can be recognized if looked for (Figs. 3–5 and 3–6). The distribution of the gas-filled loops, if asymmetrical, may suggest retroperitoneal tumor or internal hernia; annular pancreas may be thought of with obstruction of the second portion of the duodenum (Fig. 3–7); stones in the ureter or compression fracture of the spine suggests adynamic ileus (Fig. 3–8); free air in the peritoneal cavity suggests a ruptured viscus and indicates surgical intervention. In cases of intussusception, a soft tissue shadow of the intussusception may be visible, at times outlined by gas.

Fig. 3–1.

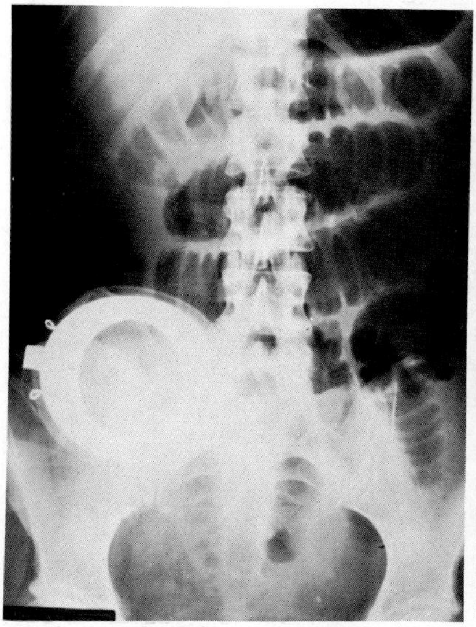

Fig. 3–2.

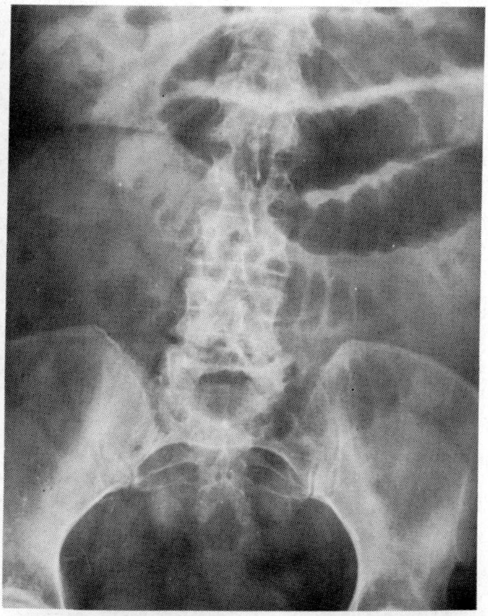

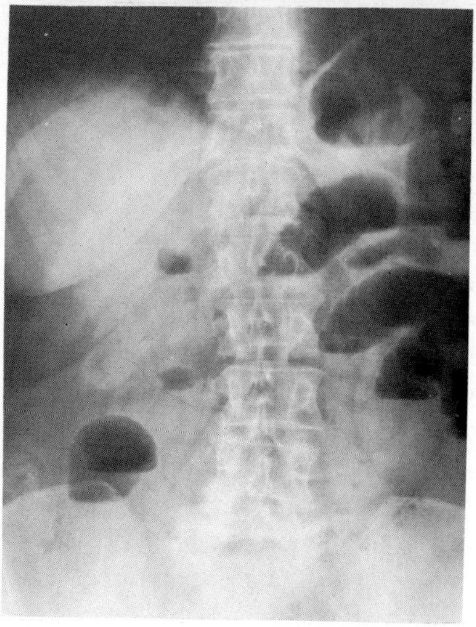

Fig. 3–3.

Figure 3–1. Plain film of abdomen. Small bowel obstructed at ileostomy. Note thickness of bowel wall between gas patterns.

Figure 3–2. Plain film of abdomen, jejunal obstruction.

Figure 3–3. Upright film of abdomen, jejunal obstruction. Note fluid levels.

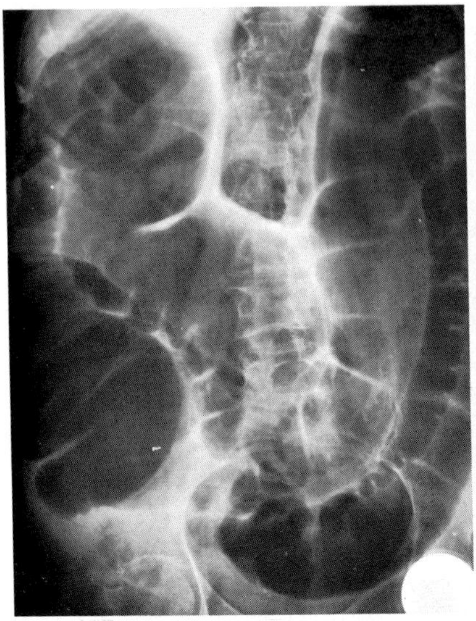

Fig. 3–4.

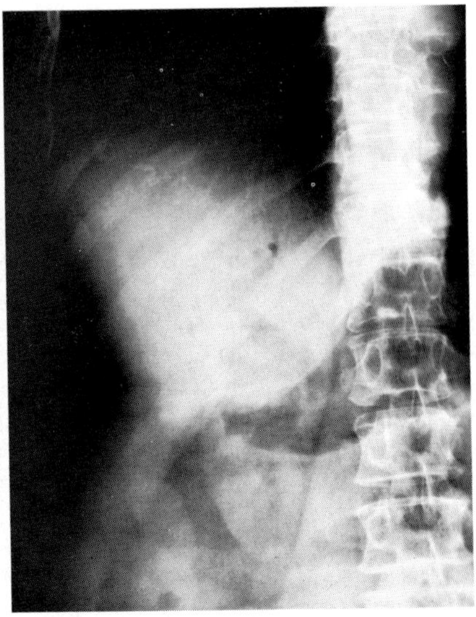

Fig. 3–5.

Figure 3–4. Plain film of abdomen. Low colonic obstruction.
Figure 3–5. "Gallstone ileus." Note air in biliary tree.

Several pitfalls in radiograph interpretation are worth emphasizing. Infants, children, and elderly and bedridden patients not infrequently have significant amounts of gas in the small intestine without obstruction. Tabes dorsalis and diabetic acidosis at times are associated with appreciable air in the small intestine that does not indicate the presence of small bowel obstruction. Conversely, gas in the colon does not mean that small bowel obstruction cannot be present in significant degree. The obstruction may be partial and allow some gas to traverse to the colon. In addition, recent enemas given in an effort to relieve obstruction can introduce large amounts of gas into the colon. Occasionally because of the large amount of fluid within obstructed loops and because of the trapping of that fluid by proximal and distal occlusion, as in volvulus, no air fluid level will be visualized in obstruction. Additionally, the air may not be visualized if only recumbent studies are obtained. It must also be kept in mind that simple mechanical obstruction may not be reflected in the plain upright roentgenogram by any intestinal gas or distention. This is a most unusual situation, however.

The development of water soluble radiopaque dyes for use in the gastrointestinal tract have aided greatly in the diagnosis of unusual obstruction.[83, 104, 105] We are reluctant to use oral barium in the presence of suspected obstruction, but frequently find use for the water soluble agents. With these one can frequently demonstrate dilated loops of bowel and failure of normal progression of dye—signs suggestive of obstruction. Or on

Fig. 3–6.

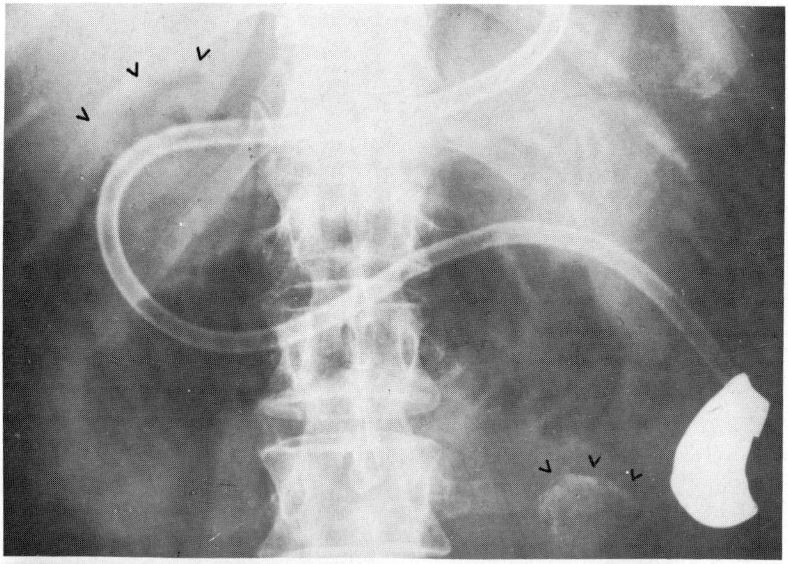

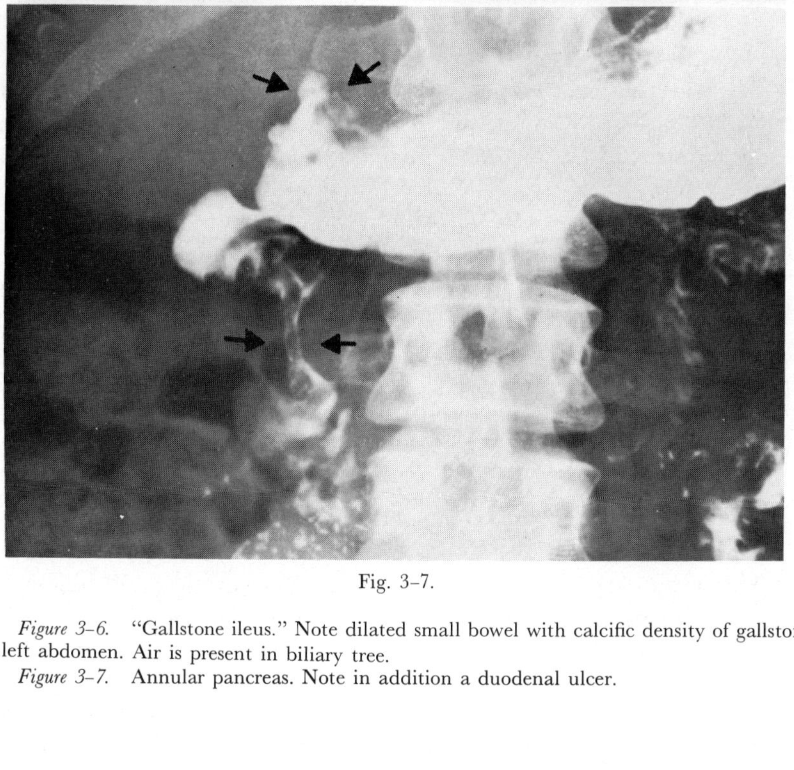

Fig. 3–7.

Figure 3–6. "Gallstone ileus." Note dilated small bowel with calcific density of gallstone in left abdomen. Air is present in biliary tree.

Figure 3–7. Annular pancreas. Note in addition a duodenal ulcer.

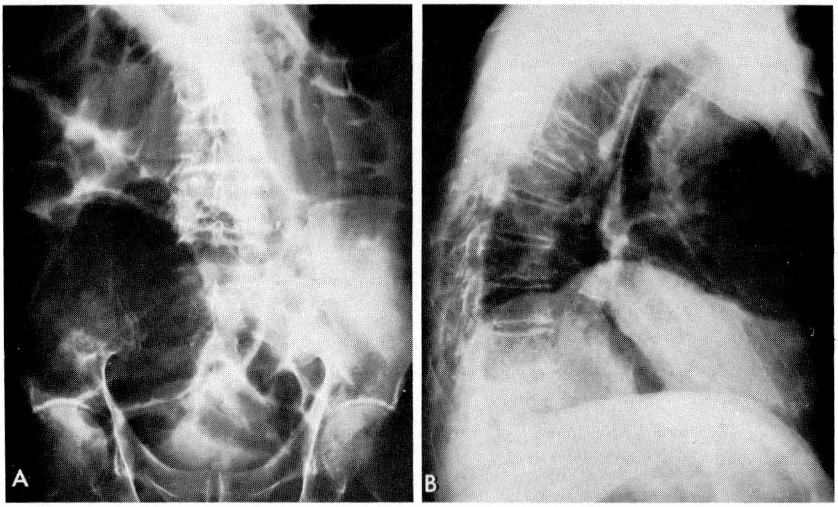

Figure 3–8. *A* and *B*, Gaseous distention of small and large bowel due to compression fracture of spine (T10).

the other hand, the distention of postoperative ileus can be identified by the normal progression of the dye through the gastrointestinal tract (Fig. 3–9*A*, *B*, *C*, *D*).

The use of a long intestinal tube as a conduit for a contrast material is often advantageous. Remarkably precise roentgenograms of obstructing or partially obstructing lesions can sometimes be obtained with this technique. When the presence of organic obstruction is in doubt, this technique often can help with the decision regarding the advisability of laparotomy or removal of the tube.

The development of contrast visualization of the branches of the abdominal aorta has implications for the early diagnosis of bowel obstruction due to arterial insufficiency. Future refinements in these techniques hold promise for development of a method of diagnosis in cases with disordered small intestinal function when suitable arterial surgery can prevent progression to the stage of intestinal obstruction and irreversible bowel necrosis.

OTHER DIAGNOSTIC PROCEDURES

Laboratory estimation of the leukocyte concentration and differential count in the peripheral blood is mandatory in following patients with obstruction. Elevation of the white count with a shift to the left of polymorphonuclear forms is evidence suggestive of bowel necrosis.

Another technique for the recognition of the presence of necrotic bowel is abdominal paracentesis with study of the peritoneal fluid so obtained.[49]

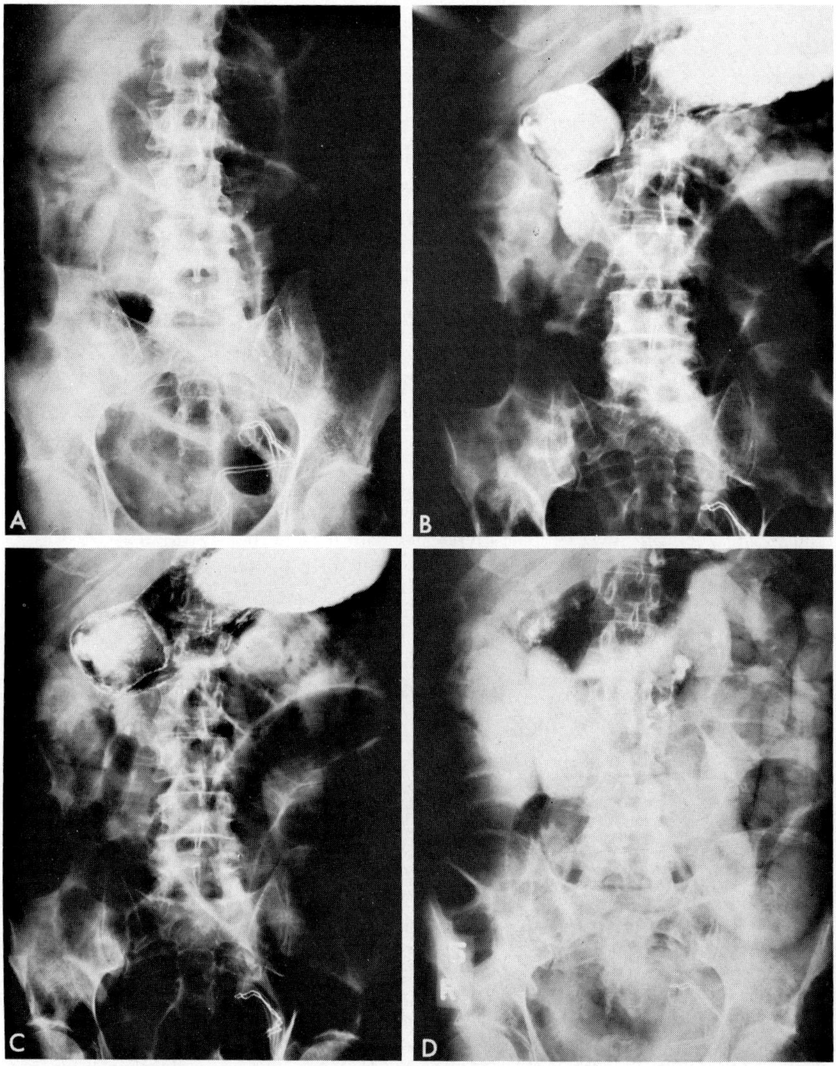

Figure 3–9. Progression of Gastrographin through bowel demonstrating postoperative ileus. *A,* Plain abdominal film. *B,* One half hour after Gastrographin given orally. *C,* Two and one half hours after Gastrographin given orally. *D,* Five hours after Gastrographin given orally.

A dark red or black fluid is pathognomonic of necrotic bowel.[78] Studies* of this fluid have shown that in the presence of necrotic intestine, the potassium concentration is much higher (in the range of 6 to 12 mEq. per liter) than that normal for extracellular fluids. Presumably this elevation of the potassium level is indicative of the release of intracellular potassium following cell death and dissolution.

* Unpublished observations of J. W. Braasch.

DIFFERENTIAL DIAGNOSIS

Four important questions must be answered by the physician who treats a patient with small bowel obstruction. These are: (1) Is intestinal obstruction present? (2) Is the obstruction due to paralytic ileus which should be treated conservatively? (3) Is there any nonviable or marginally viable bowel present? (4) What is the location and the cause of the obstruction?

Usually the diagnosis of intestinal obstruction is not difficult. Occasionally, however, the differential diagnosis between obstruction and severe gastroenteritis, lead colic, porphyria, sickle cell anemia, tabes dorsalis, or severe psychoneurosis with aerophagia or nongaseous bloating[3] can be obscure. The following is a case in point.

A 24-year-old female was admitted with crampy abdominal pain, nausea, vomiting, abdominal distention, and abdominal tenderness. She had had no bowel movement for four days. She gave a history of having had 12 laparotomies for intestinal obstruction. Roentgenograms of the abdomen showed dilated loops of small intestine (Fig. 3–10). The presence of air in the colon could not be relied upon to rule out a partial obstruction. A water soluble radiopaque dye (Gastrographin) was given by Levin tube, and serial films demonstrated its rapid course to the terminal colon (Fig. 3–11). On this basis the diagnosis of aerophagia was made and laparotomy was avoided.

The second question related to the differential diagnosis of mechanical obstruction and paralytic ileus is often not easily answered.[86] Of aid in the

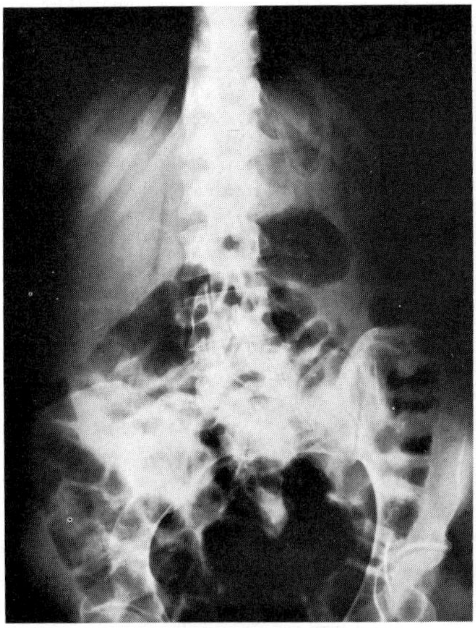

Fig. 3–10.

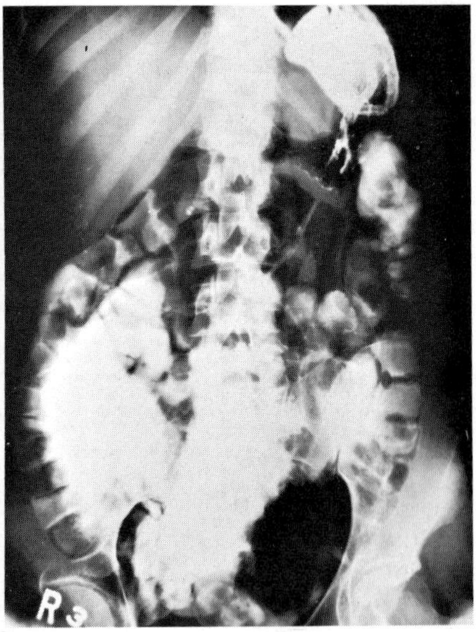

Fig. 3–11.

Figure 3–10. Plain film of abdomen demonstrating the results of aerophagia.
Figure 3–11. Three hours after Gastrographin administration in the same patient.

differential diagnosis is the presence of crampy abdominal pain, which is more often associated with mechanical obstruction.[31] The presence of conditions which have been known to be associated with paralytic ileus should be noted. These include ureteral calculus, common duct calculi with colic, compression fracture (Fig. 3–8*A* and *B*) of the lumbar or lower thoracic spine, acute appendicitis, perforated peptic ulcer, torsion of ovarian cyst, peritonitis, pancreatitis, recent laparotomy, repair of ventral hernia, pneumonitis, dissecting aneurysm, pulmonary infarct, and others. In the presence of these conditions, the demonstration of air throughout the large and small intestinal tract implies the presence of paralytic ileus.

The recognition of the presence of nonviable bowel can be difficult.[13, 92, 94, 104] Even in centers where great interest is taken in intestinal obstruction, the rate of failure of early recognition of strangulated obstruction can be as high as 21 to 25 percent.[94, 96, 109] Welch[109] has surveyed the opinions in the literature on this point and observes that it is common for the temperature to be high, the pulse rate to be markedly elevated, tenderness and palpable mass to be found, and the white count to be over 15,000 in strangulated obstruction. Conversely, he also points out that these observations are at times made in cases of simple obstruction, and therefore cannot be used as an infallible guide to the presence of necrotic bowel.

TREATMENT OF SMALL INTESTINAL OBSTRUCTION

GENERAL APPROACH AND TIMING OF OPERATION

In no other field in the practice of abdominal surgery is our heritage of past experience more helpful than in the management of the patient with an acutely obstructed small intestine.[2] The decision for and the timing of operative intervention is of vital importance when, as often, a life is at stake. In all cases of small intestinal obstruction, strenuous attempts should be made to restore toward normal the abnormalities associated with obstruction. These include gastric and small bowel distention, blood volume deficiency, deficits in water and certain electrolytes, and abnormalities in the cardiorespiratory or renal systems. The prophylaxis or treatment of infection should not be neglected. While these measures aimed at restitution of the body economy are being planned and carried out, consideration is given to the appropriateness of surgical treatment. Laparotomy is urgent in any case in which nonviable or marginally viable bowel is suspected. Gastric and small bowel decompression and the restorative ancillary procedures mentioned previously should not be prolonged beyond one or two hours under these circumstances. A current postoperative mortality in cases of strangulated obstruction of 20 to 40 percent[92, 94, 96] emphasizes the urgency of operative treatment in these cases. In the absence of findings suggesting impaired circulation to a loop of bowel, operative treatment can be delayed and efforts at long tube decompression of the intestine initiated unless contraindicated for other reasons. Especially in early postoperative obstruction or in recurrent obstruction due to adhesions and bands, delay in operative intervention is recommended. However, if the obstruction persists and the long tube fails to enter the duodenum and jejunum, fruitless attempts at intubation should be abandoned and laparotomy should be carried out. In a case of acute obstruction which has persisted for two or three days, even without evidence of nonviable bowel, laparotomy should be carried out. Bollinger and Fowler[17] have reported a sharply rising mortality rate even in obstruction without strangulation prolonged beyond one or two days.

In summary, the best clinical approach to acute small intestinal obstruction is surgical. However, the mortality is lessened and the operating conditions improved if the patients' intra- and extracellular fluid components are restored to normal and the bowel is deflated prior to operative intervention. Under certain conditions, delay in surgical treatment is advisable; these include reasonable doubt as to the existence of mechanical obstruction, relenting obstruction, a history of multiple recurrent obstructions, obstructions in the postoperative period, obstructions due to inflammatory intra-abdominal conditions, and obstructions due to abdominal carcinomatosis. Under other conditions, surgical treatment is advisable after a delay measured in hours or no more than one or two days.

FLUID AND ELECTROLYTE REPLACEMENT

Clinical estimations of the quality and quantity of fluid lost in small bowel obstruction are frequently possible.[13, 76] Loss of chloride is out of proportion to sodium in high obstructions and approximately equal to sodium in lower small intestinal obstructions. Fluids lost due to vomiting or suction contain potassium and magnesium,[59] so replacement of these ions is also advisable. With an obstructive course measured in days, total losses can be extensive. The dilated small bowel obstructed in its lower portion can accommodate several liters of fluid that has been effectively removed from the circulation. The correction of deficits producing tachycardia, hypotension, oliguria, and stupor can entail the infusion of many liters of fluid. Guidelines for the estimation of the total fluid needed have been given by Roberts et al.[91] A variety of types of infusion fluid are available and include those of balanced salt content as in normal saline or hypertonic salt solutions, sodium-rich solutions containing sodium bicarbonate, and chloride-rich solutions containing ammonium chloride. Chemical estimations of plasma sodium, chloride, potassium, carbon dioxide, and pH should be used in planning and carrying out restitution. The clinical response of the blood pressure, pulse rate, urinary output, and mentation should be closely followed. The use of plasma volume and blood volume expanders such as albumin solutions, dextran, and whole blood should not be neglected when indicated.

Tube Decompression

Since the original use of duodenal or gastric decompression in obstruction by Westerman,[110] and the exploitation of this technique by Levin,[60] Wangensteen,[107] and Miller and Abbott,[73] some of the methods of intubation have become quite sophisticated. To overcome the universal difficulty in passing these tubes into the upper jejunum, various techniques have been described.[13] The use of magnetic guidance[55] or wire stylet manipulation[95] has been advocated. However, such techniques have not been universally accepted because of failure to readily reproduce these authors' successes.

For an exhaustive summary of the types of tubes available, the techniques of intubation, and the complications of tube decompression, the reader is referred to a monograph on bowel obstruction by Cantor and Reynolds.[24] Generally, usage is restricted to the tubes shown in Figure 3–12. The techniques of passage of such tubes into the upper jejunum are well known and involve the use of a weighted tip and appropriate positioning of the patient so that the tube negotiates the desired course through the pylorus and duodenum. In spite of published data showing a high success rate of passage, many surgeons including the authors have experienced considerable difficulty in passing these long tubes into the jejunum in obstructed patients. Persistence in attempts to pass such a tube in the face of repeated failures is not recommended. It is much better to settle for gastric decompression with either a Levin or long tube followed by laparotomy. In cases of continuing obstruction, even if successful decompression of the distended small bowel is accomplished, laparotomy should not usually be long delayed, and the surgeon should look on long tube decompression as no more than an aid to surgery.

Our preference as to type of long tube employed is the Cantor tube pictured in Figure 3–12.[23] This tube has the advantage of a large lumen for decompression.

It is usually advisable to leave the long tube in the stomach if its passage into the jejunum or duodenum is unsuccessful. At laparotomy the tube can frequently be advanced into the desired position. As an aid in accomplishing this, a stab wound can be made in the jejunum near the ligament of Treitz and a long curved instrument passed to grasp and advance the tip of the long tube. Advancement further in the small intestine can be accomplished by milking the distended balloon. The use of a long coiled spring tube for operative decompression, inserted through the patient's nose and manipulated from the head of the table, has been advised.[58]

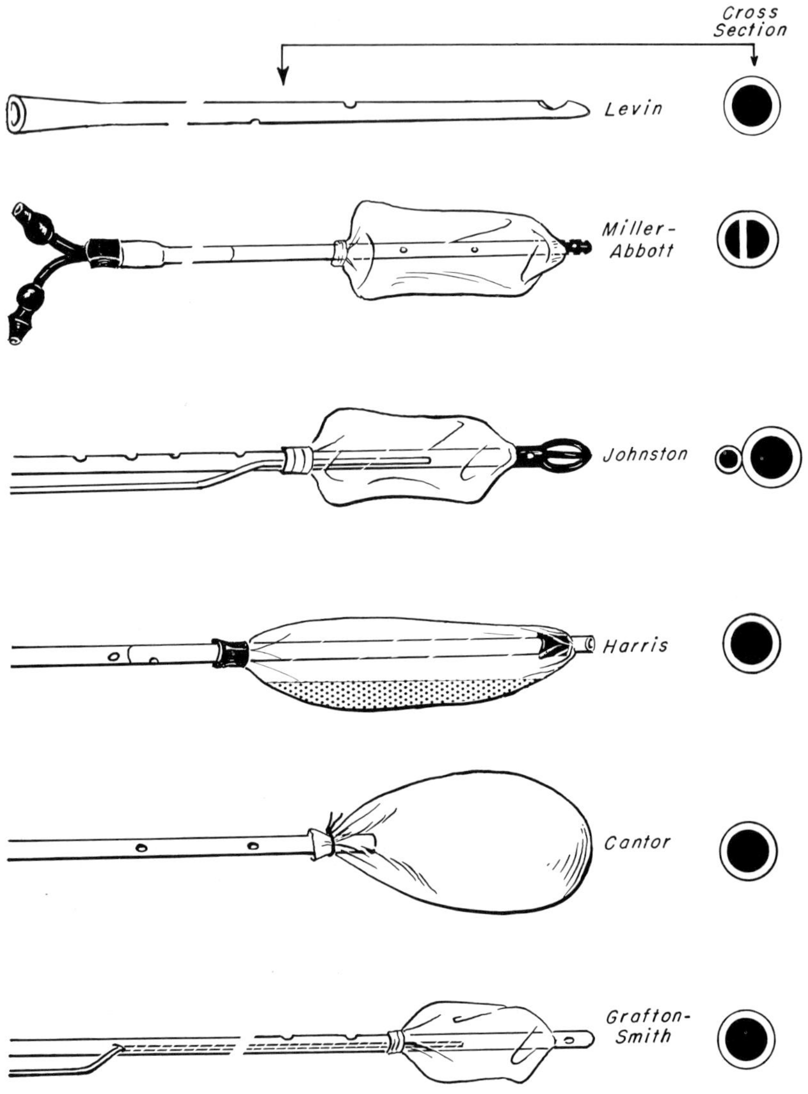

Figure 3–12. Types of gastrointestinal tubes used in decompression. (From Welch, C. E.: Intestinal Obstruction. Chicago, Year Book Medical Publishers, Inc., 1958, p. 108.)

INTESTINAL PACING

Following the development of cardiac pacemakers, the concept of intestinal pacing has been explored by Bilgutay et al.[14] The so-called paralytic ileus which follows abdominal operation or spinal fracture is characterized by a dilated bowel without tone or effective peristalsis. It seemed attractive to try to stimulate the smooth muscle fibers of the upper gastrointestinal tract in the hope of increasing propulsive peristaltic activity. This has been accomplished with an electrode introduced into the gastric antrum and reported to be effective in patients with postoperative ileus and ileus following a renal colic.[14] These authors suggested that earlier alimentation and shorter periods of gastrointestinal suction resulted. Another group has attempted to confirm Bilgutay's results without success.[87] As yet this concept and technique have not received extensive trial.

SURGICAL CONSIDERATIONS

One of the hazards of surgical intervention in cases of intestinal obstruction is aspiration of gastric contents, especially in the induction and awakening phases of general anesthesia. It is therefore of vital importance to be certain of gastric decompression by tube aspiration. The use of spinal anesthesia is a way of avoiding this sometimes fatal possibility. However, this type of anesthesia can be accompanied by serious episodes of hypotension and for this reason is at times undesirable in the seriously ill patient. Local infiltration, or field block anesthesia, if skillfully given, can be used to great advantage, especially in thin elderly patients. Not only can the procedure proceed without difficulties in exposure, but the risks of the hypotension of spinal anesthesia and those others associated with general anesthesia can be avoided. However, general anesthesia supplemented by the use of muscle relaxants is usually chosen. The early introduction of a cuffed intratracheal tube to avoid problems with aspiration is advisable.

Frequently, the exact site of obstruction is not known. Under these circumstances the incision should be made in such a way that it can be easily extended to give access to a distant area of the abdomen. A vertical abdominal incision fulfills these qualifications. If it is seen, following inspection of the problem with the abdomen opened, that easy access is not afforded without extension of the incision to excessive lengths, it is usually preferable to close the initial incision and make a more suitable approach.

At times the site and nature of the obstruction are known to the operator either because of characteristics of the history, physical findings, or roentgenograms of the abdomen. In these instances, a transverse incision is entirely acceptable and to some operators preferable. In the case of postoperative obstruction in which there is no doubt as to the integrity of the original incision, it is our practice to make the second incision elsewhere, avoiding reopening the initial incision and the risk of postoperative hernia at that site. This second incision must be placed so that tissue between the two is not compromised.

In general, the surgeon should allow himself generous working room for total intraabdominal exploration as there are numerous cases in which a secondary lesion has been missed because of inadequate exposure.

Of extreme importance are the initial observations of the intraabdominal contents on opening the peritoneum. If dilated and collapsed bowel are seen, one can be sure of the diagnosis of obstruction, and the cause must be found. Frequently loops of distended bowel hinder exploration. After preliminary observations it is often helpful to decompress these distended loops by enterotomy.[5, 66] We prefer a Poole suction tip for this purpose (Fig. 3-13).[74] This instrument can be introduced through a small stab wound in the bowel and advanced in either direction, using the plunger type suction control, reefing the bowel over the instrument. In such a way the entire small intestine can be emptied easily through two stab wounds without spillage.

Other aids in operative diagnosis and treatment include the proper positioning of the operating table so that small bowel and omentum do not obscure the field. Partial or total evisceration of the loops of small intestine can be used for the same purpose.

Not infrequently the surgeon must judge the viability of a strangulated segment of small intestine. If the normal pink color and the peristaltic action return to a loop of intestine after release of obstruction to its vascular supply, there is no problem with this decision. At times it is advisable to wrap the bowel in question in warm saline pads and wait for a 10-minute period

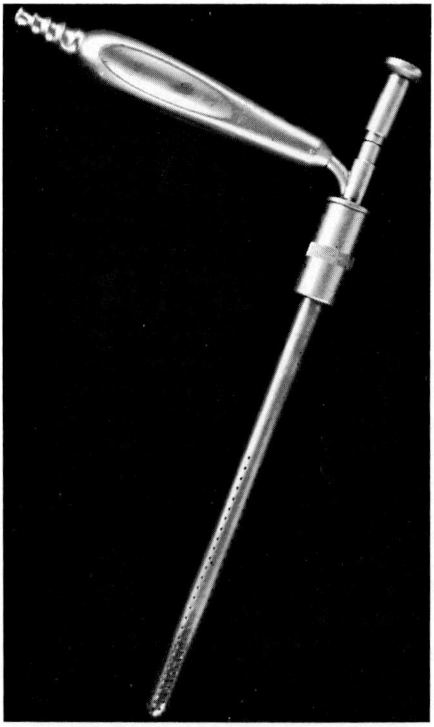

Figure 3–13. Poole suction tip for operative decompression of distended bowel.

to judge the return of normal color. If there is doubt in the operator's mind as to the viability of the loop, it is far safer to resect and perform an end-to-end anastomosis.

SPECIFIC CAUSES OF OBSTRUCTION

Adhesive Obstruction

The most common cause of small bowel obstruction is adhesive obstruction.[30, 32] Formerly hernial obstruction was more common, but as the frequency of elective hernia repair has increased, hernial obstruction has decreased. Adhesive obstruction generally is preceded by abdominal surgery. Less commonly the obstructing bands and adhesions are congenital,[106] associated with a Meckel's diverticulum or intraabdominal abscess, or are secondary to abdominal trauma. It has been estimated that there has been no previous abdominal surgery in 5 to 10 percent of cases.

In view of this incidence, the prevention of postoperative adhesions assumes vital importance and must be considered during every intra-abdominal procedure.[19, 33, 106] The covering of raw surfaces which have been denuded of peritoneum is well advised and should include the closure by suturing of retroperitoneal surfaces after colon resection and the covering of sites of removal of pelvic organs and raw areas on the surface of bowel. The avoidance of talcum powder granulomas by the substitution of starch powder has aided greatly in the prevention of adhesive obstruction due to talc.[62] It is recognized that starch powder is not entirely innocuous in this regard, and care in glove cleansing should be taken regardless of the type of powder used. The availability of a semiliquid lubricant markedly reduces the need for a powder.

The use of various drugs or substances for parenteral use or direct application to the peritoneal cavity to prevent adhesions has not received wide clinical usage.[19, 22, 33] Reliance should, therefore, be placed on prevention of adhesions by meticulous surgical technique.

The treatment of established adhesive obstruction includes fluid and electrolyte replacement and tube decompression. Operative intervention is recommended in most cases since permanent remission without operation is unusual and the differential diagnosis of adhesive obstruction from other causative mechanisms and from strangulated obstruction can be difficult.[11, 69] Thus, a clinical trial of tube suction could be carried out for 24 to 48 hours, but laparotomy should be performed in the absence of definite clinical improvement at the end of this time. It is axiomatic that laparotomy should be immediate if there are signs and symptoms of peritoneal irritation.

The operative armamentarium includes lysis of adhesions, the freeing of matted loops of bowel, the release of abnormal fixation of the small bowel, the removal of omentum, and the resection of nonviable intestine or of intestine severely damaged by dissection. A resection which removes enough bowel to impair absorption is to be avoided at almost all costs.

A major problem in the treatment of adhesive obstruction is encountered in that patient who has had repetitive small bowel obstruction and multiple operative procedures for its relief. In fact, in these situations the diagnosis of obstruction can be most difficult. Plain and upright films of the abdomen are often not diagnostic, since with partial obstruction air can be seen throughout the gastrointestinal tract. Similarly, patients of a highly neurotic temperament who are "air swallowers" can present with extreme abdominal distention, crampy abdominal pain, nausea and vomiting, and distention of the small bowel with occasional fluid levels. Of aid in this dilemma is a barium or Gastrographin meal and great persistence with conservative management.

If laparotomy is carried out in patients with multiple recurrences of obstruction, removal of the omentum should be considered if this structure is markedly involved in the adhesive process. The small bowel intestinal plication procedure or its many variants should be considered.[80, 85] These procedures involve the planned arrangement of the loops of small intestine so that when adhesive binding takes place in the postoperative period, obstructing intestinal kinks will be prevented. Figure 3–14 depicts the placement of sutures to appose the loops in gentle curves to accomplish

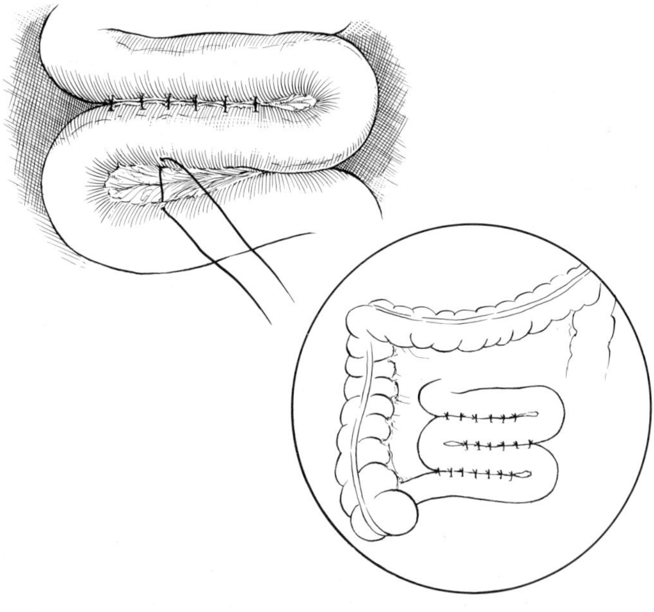

Figure 3–14. Placement of sutures in plication procedure.

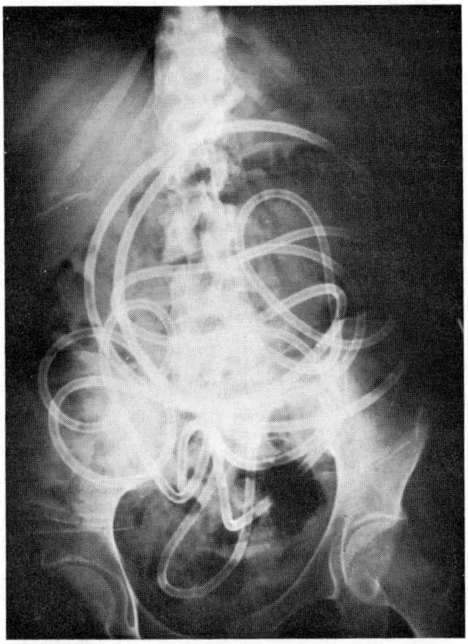

Figure 3–15. Abdominal roentgenogram showing long intestinal tube used as a splint in jejunum and ileum.

this purpose. A substantial morbidity and mortality follow this procedure to include death, 5 percent; obstruction, 6 percent; and fistulas, 5 percent.[112]

As an alternative to this procedure, the placement of a long intestinal tube through the jejunum and ileum through a small jejunostomy incision sutured to the lateral abdominal wall has much to recommend it.[68, 111] This tube is left in place during the three- or four-week postoperative period (Fig. 3–15) when adhesions are formed. The gentle curves of the tube in the bowel stabilize the small intestine during this time.

Sidetracking operations are not recommended in the treatment of recurrent obstruction. The creation of bypassed loops which can still be partially obstructed and which have the undesirable features of blind loops should be avoided.

Hernial Obstruction

Rivaling adhesive obstruction in frequency is obstruction due to fixation of the small bowel in hernial sacs or orifices. A working classification of hernias which have been known to be implicated in small bowel obstruction is shown in Table 3–3, adapted from Welch.[109]

Of this extensive list, inguinal, femoral, and umbilical hernias are the most common sites of small intestinal incarceration, and these areas should be included in the physical examination of any patient with small intestinal obstruction. Because of the location of these hernias within the abdominal wall with their contents sealed off and isolated from the peritoneal

Table 3–3. Classification of Hernias Implicated With Small Intestinal Obstruction*

I. Extraabdominal (external)
    A. Inguinal
        1. Indirect
        2. Direct
        3. Combined indirect and direct
        4. Sliding
    B. Femoral
    C. Umbilical
    D. Epigastric
    E. Ventral
        1. Spontaneous
        2. Acquired
    F. Diaphragmatic
        1. Acquired-caval or aortic hiatus hernia
        2. Congenital
            a. Absence of diaphragm
            b. Pleuroperitoneal
            c. Foramen of Morgagni
        3. Traumatic
    G. Interstitial (properitoneal, intramuscular, inguinosuperficial, external supravesical)
    H. Prevesical (internal supravesical)
    I. Lumbar
    J. Obturator
    K. Sciatic
    L. Perineal
    M. Richter's
    N. Littre's
    O. Appendiceal
II. Intraabdominal (internal)
    A. Anomalous fossa
        1. Paraduodenal
        2. Paracecal
        3. Intersigmoid
        4. Foramen of Winslow
    B. Anomalous opening
        1. Mesenteric
        2. Omental
        3. Broad ligament
    C. Postoperative
        1. About gastroenterostomy stoma
        2. Behind enterocolic anastomosis
        3. About ileostomy or colostomy stoma
        4. Through operative defect
            a. Mesenteric trap
            b. Defect in omentum
            c. Trap left from uterine suspension
            d. Defect in pelvic floor

*Adapted from Welch, C. E.: Intestinal Obstruction. Chicago, Year Book Medical Publishers, Inc., 1958. Used by permission of Year Book Medical Publishers, Inc., pp. 239–240.

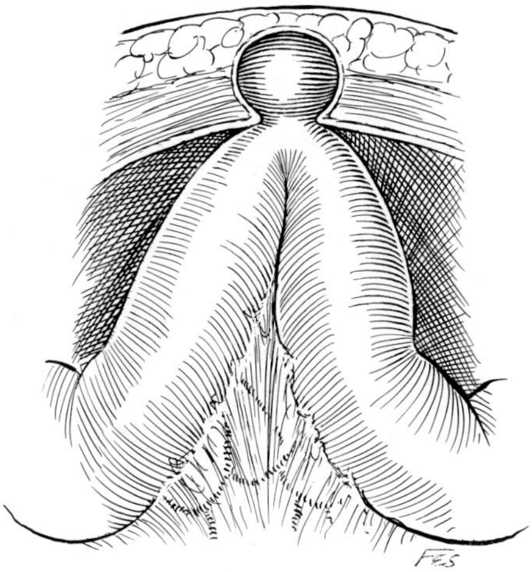

Figure 3–16. Richter's hernia.

cavity, the diagnosis of infarction of the bowel can at times be difficult and this complication can be far advanced when recognized.

Forceful reduction of incarcerated external hernias is to be deplored. Rupture of loops of bowel, reduction of gangrenous bowel, and reduction of the hernial ring and bowel have been known under these circumstances.

The entity of Richter's hernia should be considered in any patient presenting with nausea, vomiting, and abdominal pain, yet without apparent intestinal obstruction as evidenced by normal bowel movements or diarrhea.[51, 89] In this situation, only a part of the wall of the bowel may be involved in a hernial ring such that there is no occlusion of the lumen of the intestine and there is no external mass in the hernial sac (Fig. 3–16).

The operative approach to an incarcerated hernia should ensure adequate exposure of the obstructing ring and in some cases abdominal exposure of the loops of bowel entering the ring. This latter feature may be desirable for resection and anastomosis in the presence of necrotic or nonviable bowel. When there is a problem regarding the advisability of resecting a questionably viable loop of intestine, the dilemma should be solved in favor of resection. An appealing technique of management of a strangulated, gangrenous femoral hernia is that of Dennis and Varco,[36] which involves an en bloc resection of the sac, the ring, and the intestine aided by wide exposure of the ring and a peritoneal incision (Fig. 3–17). In repairing femoral hernias in cases with viable small bowel, the McVay repair is preferred.[71] The usual oblique inguinal incision can be T'd and the inguinal ligament severed.

External hernias in other locations are uncommon, but when they do occur they are characterized by a high incidence of strangulation usually due to their late recognition. Figure 3–18 illustrates their position. Koontz[52] has reviewed some of these rarer hernias comprehensively.

Delayed obstruction of the small bowel occasionally occurs after reduction and is due to the formation of a stricture of the bowel at the site of

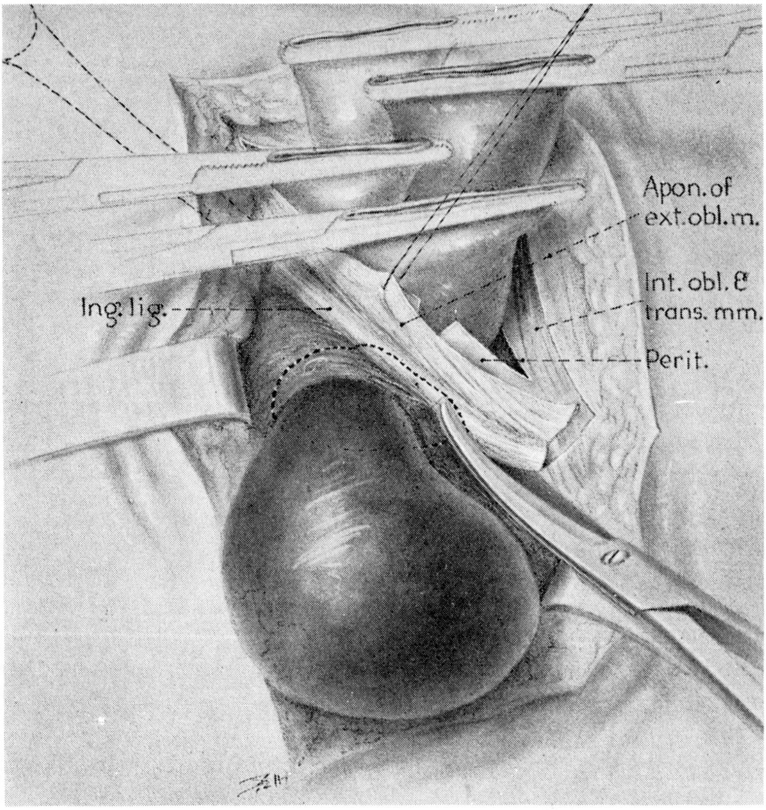

Figure 3–17. Repair of gangrenous femoral hernia. (From Dennis, C., and Varco, R. L.: Surgery *22:*315, August, 1947.)

impingement of the hernial ring.[10] This should be recognized as a definite entity; bypass or resection is indicated.

Anomalies of intestinal fixation are manifest by improper fusion to the retroperitoneal parieties.[21, 106] As illustrated in Figure 3–19, posterior fusion failure of the mesentery of the descending colon leaves a potential space posterior to this mesentery which communicates with the general peritoneal cavity just under the inferior mesenteric vein. Similarly, a potential space exists under the hepatic flexure and duodenum.

Recognition of incarceration in such hernias can be difficult, but is possible in some cases because of the localization of multiple air-filled loops to the right or left of the midline. In repairing such hernias, care must be taken that the inferior mesenteric vein or the middle colic artery is not injured as it courses along the free edge of the mesentery.

Other anomalous fossae include those around the cecum and adjacent to the sigmoid colon. Additional potential and actual hernial rings can be found in the mesentery,[74] omentum, or the broad ligaments. Occasionally

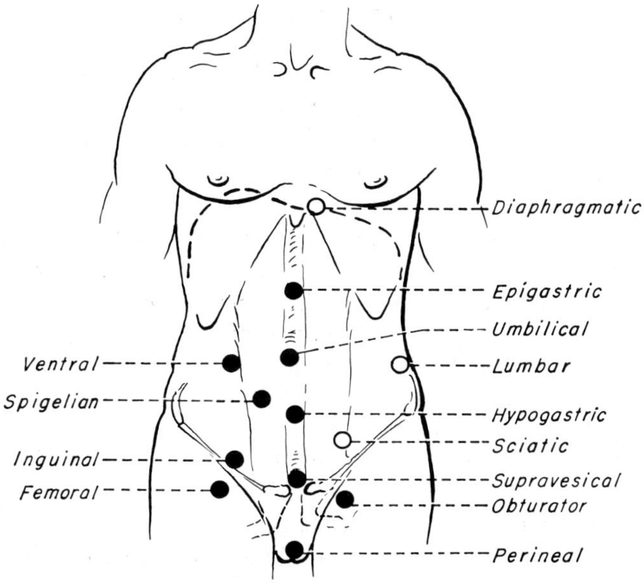

Figure 3–18. Position of external hernias. (From Welch, C. E.: Intestinal Obstruction. Chicago, Year Book Medical Publishers, Inc., 1958, p. 241.)

small bowel has been known to herniate through the foramen of Winslow. Other intraabdominal hernias are listed in Table 3–3. Of major importance in considering such herniations is the realization that such hernias are extremely difficult to recognize. Prompt surgical relief is imperative, as spontaneous reduction is unlikely and the chance of strangulation is high. Langley,[54] Harrison and Cheek,[47] Venner,[103] May and Brintnall,[67] Bowles,[18] and Baron[9] have reported on these rarer intraabdominal hernias.

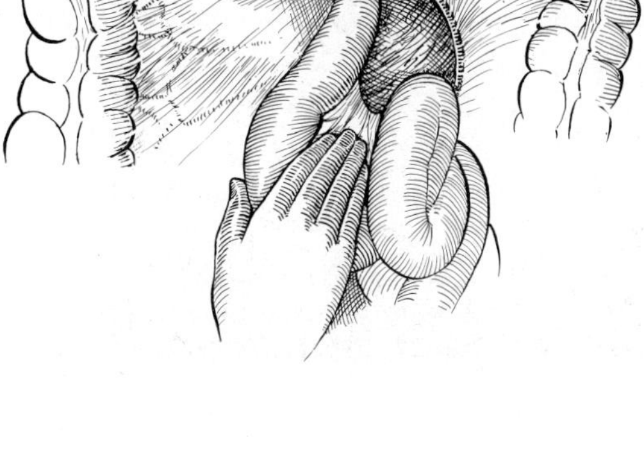

Figure 3–19. Paraduodenal hernia due to failure of fusion of descending colon mesentery. Note position of inferior mesenteric vein.

OBTURATION OBSTRUCTION

As a group, obstruction of the small intestine by an intraluminal foreign body is rare,[25, 35, 81] but one mechanism, gallstone obstruction, is a popular subject for surgical review.[64, 75] So-called gallstone ileus is caused by the impingement of a large gallstone, usually at a point of narrowing in the small intestine. Frequently, the patient has been unaware of the development of gallstones or of the cholecystoenteric fistula. Thus, the first symptoms experienced will be those of small bowel obstruction. The most common site of lodgment of the stone is the narrowed terminal ileum, usually at the ileocecal valve, but one must be aware of the approximately 30 percent incidence of lodgment in the jejunum. The plain radiograph of the intestine is often diagnostic (Figs. 3–5 and 3–6). The cardinal signs are air in the biliary tree and small bowel obstruction proximal to a calcific density in the right lower quadrant or in the left abdomen. Figure 3–20 shows an unusual choledochoduodenal fistula with the stone in the proximal duodenum and barium outlining the biliary tree.

As recorded in the earlier literature, the operative mortality in treatment of this condition was appreciable.[70] Of late years, however, this high risk has been improved.[43] Of importance in the surgical treatment of this condition is the dislodgment of the stone proximally from its obstructing position. If it cannot be fragmented easily by external manipulation, then it must be extracted through a short enterotomy incision placed well away from the point of obstruction and in relatively normal bowel. One must also bear in mind the possibility that two or more obstructing stones or fragments may be located in the small bowel, and the intestine must be thoroughly examined for them. The presence of faceted or fractured stones

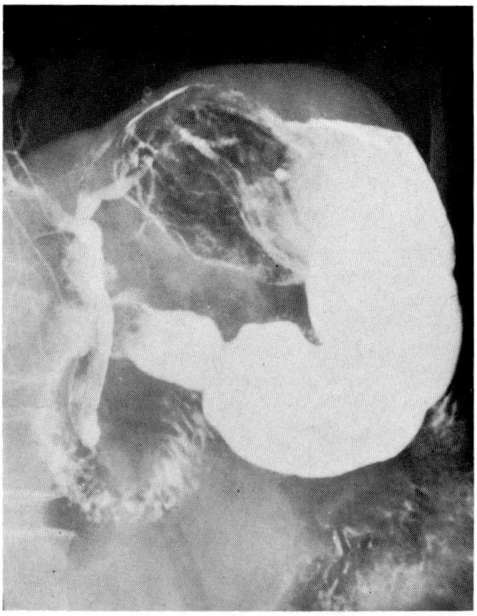

Figure 3–20. Choledochoduodenal fistula with large calculus in proximal duodenum and barium in biliary tree.

Table 3–4. Causes of Obturation Obstruction of the Small Intestine*

Gallstones
Bezoars
Trichobezoars (hair)
Phytobezoars (vegetable)
Persimmon
Other
Food boluses
Foreign bodies
Enteroliths
Worms
Meconium
Intestinal tube balloons

*Adapted from Welch, C. E.: Intestinal Obstruction. Chicago, Year Book Medical Publishers, Inc., 1958, p. 50. Used by permission of Year Book Medical Publishers, Inc.

indicates a greater likelihood of there being other undiscovered stones. Finally the gallbladder and fistula should be examined carefully for more potentially dangerous calculi. If it is evident that there are no stones in the gallbladder or fistula, it is advisable to leave the biliary tract alone. There is a small group of patients who have been followed for an appreciable time after operative relief of gallstone obstruction who have never had an operative attack on the biliary tract and who have remained well.[43] It seems reasonable to advise subsequent cholecystectomy only in those patients with a relatively long life expectancy and in whom residual calculi are suspected. At times because of long-standing pressure from the stone, a portion of the bowel will be necrotic or marginally viable. A resection of this segment is mandatory under these circumstances.

There are many other causes of obturation obstruction which are listed in Table 3–4. Figure 3–21*A* and *B* illustrates a rare grass bezoar causing small bowel obstruction. There treatment is similar to that for gallstone obstruction.[81]

ADULT INTUSSUSCEPTION

Intussusception[20, 38] occurs much less frequently in adults than in children. It has been estimated that only 5 percent of intussusceptions occur in the adult group. Frequently in adults, but not in children, there is a diverticulum or tumor that serves as a leading point for the intussusception. Thus, the treatment of adult intussusception is generally resection of the involved segment. This is urged even though no tumor or other cause is found by the surgeon because the involved edematous bowel makes accurate palpation difficult.

Intussusception in adults may be recurrent and may be associated with mild or chronic symptoms of obstruction as opposed to the acute nature of the condition in children. Two thirds of the cases will involve the small

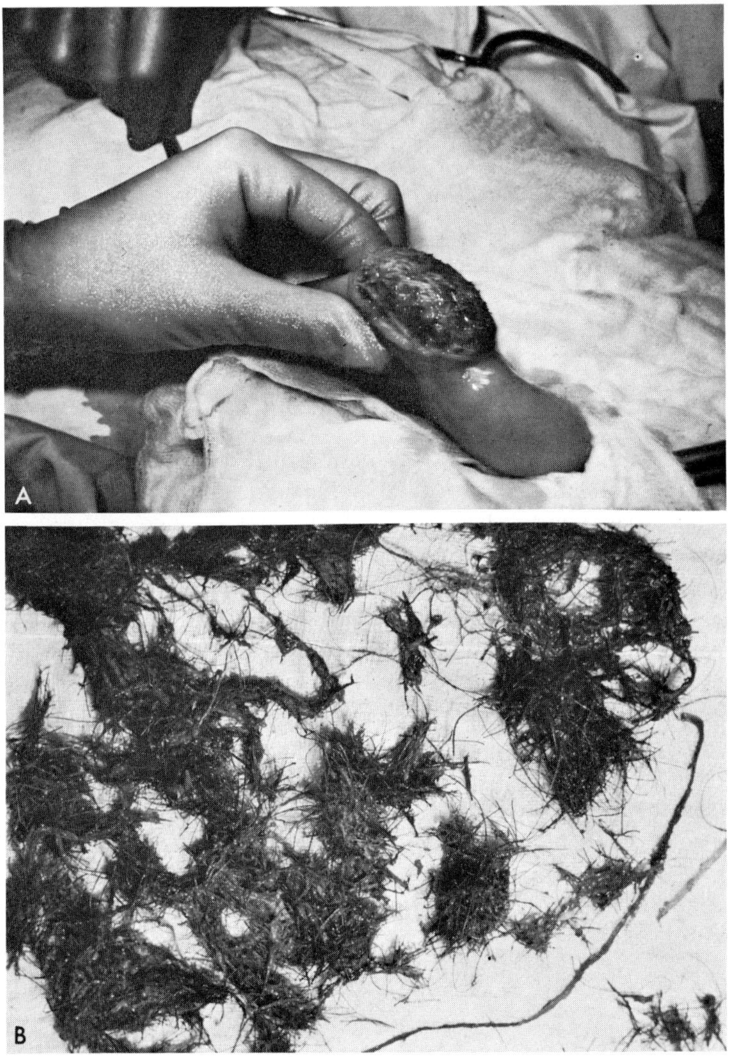

Figure 3–21. Grass bezoar causing small bowel obstruction. *A,* Removal at surgery. *B,* Contents of bezoar. (From Kune, G. A.: Brit. J. Clin. Practice *19:*217–218, April, 1965.)

intestine as well as other portions of the gastrointestinal tract. In one third just the small intestine is involved. In one large series the intussusception was associated with a malignant tumor in 60 percent and a benign tumor in 18 percent.[34] It was without apparent cause in 13 percent.

Rarer types of intussusception include jejunogastric following gastrectomy or an ileal intussusception with a Meckel's diverticulum as a leading point.[46]

VOLVULUS

Volvulus of the small intestine is one third as common as volvulus involving the colon.[90] When it does occur it is usually associated with another abnormality that serves as a fixed point about which the loops of bowel twist. In the adult these other abnormalities include Meckel's diverticulum, neoplasm, ileostomy, colostomy, adhesions or bands, or malfixation of the mesentery of the midgut.[106]

Early operation is of extreme importance in the treatment of this condition, as gangrene develops quickly following most twists. Resection of the involved bowel is usually indicated. In those cases reported by Ripstein and Miller[90] there was a postoperative mortality in excess of 50 percent if the patient came to surgery more than 12 hours after the onset of the volvulus.

EXTERNAL COMPRESSION OBSTRUCTION

Obstruction of the small bowel by carcinomatosis is relatively frequent. While isolated or localized areas occasionally are encountered causing major obstruction, the situation of widespread disease with multiple points of obstruction is more common. In the former instance localized resection or lysis of obstructing attachments is frequently worthwhile, especially in cases with slow-growing tumors. Months and even years of palliation can be achieved in these instances. It is important to cover any irremovable mass of carcinoma with omentum to prevent early recurrence of obstruction at the same site. It is, however, well known to most surgeons that with multiple point obstruction from neoplasia, attempts at extensive surgical treatment are doomed to failure and the procedure should be terminated as soon as the situation is realized.

Occasionally intraperitoneal abscesses cause small bowel obstruction by virtue of their proximity to the small intestine or by their pressure on its wall. Drainage of the abscess and bypass, lysis, or both, of the attachment are indicated if a brief trial of conservative therapy fails.

Any delayed postoperative obstruction should bring to mind the possibility of a retained foreign body. Usually the plain roentgenogram of the abdomen will reveal the obstructing instrument or sponge and indicate laparotomy.

Other rare causes of external compression obstruction include endometriosis,[29] retroperitoneal tumors, mesenteric cysts and tumors, and wandering spleen.[1]

DUODENAL OBSTRUCTION

The causes of obstruction of the duodenum are in general unique to this particular portion of the small intestine. Because the duodenum is a retroperitoneal organ it is relatively immune from acute obstruction and strangu-

Table 3–5. Classification of Causes of Duodenal Obstruction

I. Intrinsic lesions
  - A. Duodenal ulcer
  - B. Neoplasms of duodenum
  - C. Inflammatory
    1. Enteritis
    2. Syphilis
    3. Tuberculosis

II. Extrinsic lesions
  - A. Adhesions and bands
  - B. Megaduodenum with arteriomesenteric compression
  - C. Annular pancreas
  - D. Duodenal diverticulum
  - E. Lesions of adjacent organs
    1. Pancreas
       Inflammation, cysts, neoplasms
    2. Right kidney
       Neoplasms, hydronephrosis
    3. Retroperitoneal neoplasms
    4. Right colon neoplasms
    5. Aortic aneurysms
    6. Liver
       Cysts, neoplasms
    7. Lymphadenopathy

III. Obturation obstruction

IV. Megaduodenum without luminal discontinuity
  - A. Neuromuscular disorders
  - B. Chronic idiopathic

V. Developmental lesions
  - A. Atresias and stenoses
  - B. Rotational anomalies

lation. Of the two most commonly observed causes of duodenal obstruction, duodenal ulcer is beyond the scope of this monograph, and neoplasms of the duodenum are discussed in another chapter. A large variety of lesions remain, all of them rare (Table 3–5).

Of the extrinsic lesions, adhesions and bands are at times found in the right upper quadrant. Kantor[50] considered most of these bands to be congenital in origin, and of the cases in his study, 11 percent were asymptomatic.

Superior Mesenteric Artery Syndrome

Among conditions associated with obstruction of the duodenum is the "superior mesenteric artery syndrome," seemingly the result of compression of the duodenum by the superior mesenteric vessels.[88] The numerous terms used to describe this and related conditions attest to the confusion surrounding this syndrome. These include duodenal ileus, megaduodenum, giant duodenum, Wilkie's syndrome, and chronic arteriomesenteric occlusion.

In the experience of this clinic,[82] this syndrome is much less common than in the published experience of Goin and Wilk,[45] which indicates one case in 300 upper gastrointestinal roentgenograms. In a five-year period (1957–1962), approximately 38,000 upper gastrointestinal roentgenograms were performed at the Lahey Clinic Foundation. Most of these patients had symptoms referable to the upper gastrointestinal tract. A diagnosis of superior mesenteric artery syndrome was made only five times in the 38,000 examinations, an incidence of 0.013 percent.

The etiology of the superior mesenteric artery syndrome is unknown. Traditionally it has been thought to be due to a mechanical obstruction by pressure from the superior mesenteric vessels as they cross the duodenum.[97] Grooving of the anterior surface of the normal duodenum has been noted on gross inspection[84] and radiographically (Fig. 3–22). Certain nonoperative measures designed to lessen the compression have been reported[101] to be effective in the treatment of this syndrome. Strong[97] and Major et al.[63] have demonstrated clinical relief of obstruction by an operative procedure that displaces the duodenum out of the acute angle formed by the superior mesenteric vessels and the aorta.

Opposed to this mechanical theory are those who believe a neuromuscular derangement to be responsible.[53] Support for this belief is gained from a report of a family with megaduodenum and megalocystis.[57] Evidence against a solely mechanical etiology is found in the report of two cases of megaduodenum in which the mesenteric vessels did not cross the duodenum since the colon was nonrotated,[77] and also from a series of cases with megaduodenum and, in addition, dilatation of the upper jejunum.[8]

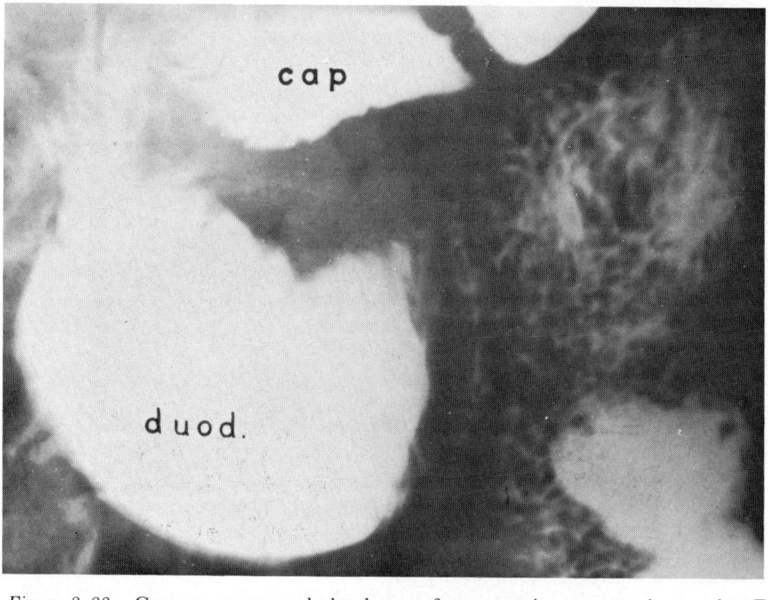

Figure 3–22. Grooves on normal duodenum from superior mesenteric vessels. (From Nugent, F. W., Braasch, J. W., and Epstein, H.: J.A.M.A. *196:*1092, June 20, 1966.)

The typical patient is a young adult, usually a woman, with an asthenic body habitus and superimposed weight loss. The symptoms of this condition are the same as those of acute or chronic high intestinal obstruction. On roentgenographic examination or inspection at surgery, dilation and hypertrophy of the first, second, and part of the third portions of the duodenum are found with retained secretions in the stomach and churning peristalsis in the duodenum. Not uncommonly in a normal study, barium is delayed temporarily where the third portion of the duodenum crosses the spine, without significant dilatation of the duodenum proximal to this point. This finding is not significant and is not accompanied by symptoms; when significant obstruction is present, the duodenum is dilated and symptoms of obstruction of the upper small bowel are present.

Table 3–6 presents some of the details of five patients with the diagnosis of superior mesenteric artery syndrome who were treated surgically by us. All these patients had symptoms of partial duodenal obstruction with nausea, occasional vomiting, anorexia, and intermittent epigastric pain and fullness. They all had noted varying amounts of weight loss coincident with or before their symptoms began.

Case 1 is an example of an advanced form of the superior mesenteric artery syndrome (Fig. 3–23). Certain features of it suggest a neuromuscular disorder of the dilated duodenum since two patent duodenojejunostomies, one of which was clearly dependent, did not adequately empty the duodenum. Duodenal biopsy in this case and duodenal and jejunal biopsy 6

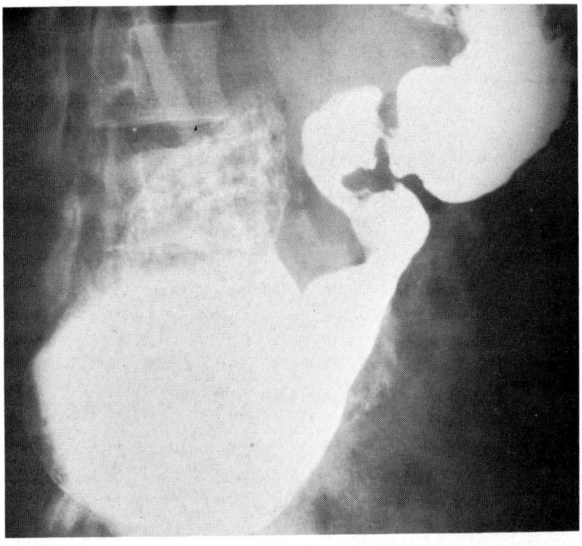

Figure 3–23. Extreme dilatation of the duodenum in case of superior mesenteric artery obstruction of duodenum. (From Nugent, F. W., Braasch, J. W., and Epstein, H.: J.A.M.A. *196:*1092, June 20, 1966.)

Table 3-6. Case Reports of Patients Who Had Surgical Treatment of Superior Mesenteric Artery Syndrome*

Case	Age and Sex	Size of duodenum	Body weight: *Before Illness*	Body weight: *Preoperatively*	Body weight: *At Follow-up*	Operation	Result	Follow-up (*years*)
1	29 M	Massively dilated	150	141	141	Duodenojejunostomy	Poor	—
				141	172	Gastric resection with gastro-jejunostomy	Excellent—good	6
2	45 F	Greatly dilated	134	130	125	Duodenojejunostomy	Excellent—good	4
3	19 M	Large	160	132	Not noted	Gastrojejunostomy	Excellent—good (immediate)	$\frac{1}{4}$
4	36 F	Markedly dilated	115	96	96	Gastrojejunostomy	Fair	4
5	57 F	Dilated	130	103	Not noted	Gastrojejunostomy; take-down ligament of Treitz	Good	1

*Adapted from Nugent, F. W., et al.: J.A.M.A. *196:*1093 (June 20) 1966.

inches from the ligament of Treitz in Case 2 showed normal myenteric plexuses. Case 1 is of further interest because the son of the patient has megalocystis and megaloureter, apparently the result of a congenital neuromuscular derangement.

The treatment for this condition is at first conservative with frequent feedings, attempts at positional relief (knee-chest), bed rest, and occasionally jejunal tube feedings. Intravenous electrolyte and blood administration should not be neglected when needed. If the conservative approach fails, laparotomy is indicated.

It is stated that the appropriate surgical treatment of this condition is duodenojejunostomy with the anastomosis placed in the dependent portion of the dilated duodenum.[6, 16, 84] Cases 1 and 2 of our series did have this anastomosis performed with variable results, whereas Cases 1, 3, 4, and 5 had a gastrojejunostomy with perhaps better results. It should be noted that the postoperative body weight did not reflect the clinical result in two cases. This series is necessarily small because of the rarity of the condition, and therefore, no definite conclusion can be reached as to the best operative procedure. We have no experience with the use of the operation proposed by Strong,[97] or severance of the ligament of Treitz, which is designed to release the terminal duodenum from its position of entrapment between the superior mesenteric vessels and the spine. If gastrojejunostomy is to be used, one would now recommend complementary vagotomy to prevent the formation of a jejunal ulcer, although vagotomy was not employed in these cases. We have seen one patient treated elsewhere by gastrojejunostomy who required reoperation because of the development of a gastrojejunal ulcer.

Annular Pancreas

Annular pancreas is a rare condition which at times causes duodenal obstruction.[26, 98] Epigastric pain, nausea, and vomiting are prominent. The diagnosis is based on an awareness of the condition and on a barium study showing narrowing of the second portion of the duodenum (Fig. 3–7). Associated peptic ulceration and duodenal atresia are not uncommon in these cases. The treatment is ideally duodenojejunostomy or, in the presence of peptic ulceration, gastric resection. Division of the encircling pancreas should not be done.

Duodenal Diverticula

Duodenal diverticula are a common finding on upper gastrointestinal barium examination; however, rarely are they symptomatic. Occasionally they, like all diverticula of the gastrointestinal tract, are subject to diverticulitis and so obstruct the adjacent duodenum. Duodenal diverticula are usually found in the second portion of the duodenum in the concave aspect of the duodenal curve near the ampulla. A more complete discussion is found in Chapter Eight.

A variety of lesions of adjacent organs has been known to obstruct the duodenum (Table 3–5).[4, 93] Obturation obstruction of the duodenum is a rare condition. Causative agents include bezoars, gallstones, and foreign bodies. Of the developmental lesions, atresias and stenoses are not discussed in this monograph on adult surgery of the small intestine, and rotational anomalies are considered in the section on hernial obstruction.

MISCELLANEOUS CAUSES OF OBSTRUCTION

Infection following appendicitis, peritonitis from other causes, paralytic ileus associated with poliomyelitis, chronic nonspecific granulomas, and retroperitoneal hemorrhage, all can cause small bowel obstruction by interfering with normal propulsive movements or by encroachment on the bowel lumen.

The subjects of mesenteric embolism and thrombosis, tumors of the small intestine, diverticulitis, nonspecific stricture and ulcer, and inflammatory lesions of the small intestine will be discussed in other chapters.

REFERENCES

1. Abell, I.: Wandering spleen with torsion of the pedicle. Ann. Surg. *98:*722–735 (Oct.) 1933.
2. Allen, A. W.: Editorial. Acute obstruction of the small intestine. Arch. Surg. *70:*476–478 (Apr.) 1955.
3. Alvarez, W. C.: Hysterical type of nongaseous abdominal bloating. Arch. Int. Med. *84:*217–245 (Aug.) 1949.
4. Baird, L. W., and Kirklin, B. R.: Obstruction of third portion of duodenum of unusual etiology; report of case. Radiology *27:*235–236 (Aug.) 1936.
5. Baker, J. W., and Ritter, K. J.: Complete surgical decompression for late obstruction of the small intestine, with reference to a method. Ann. Surg. *157:*759–769 (May) 1963.
6. Barker, L. F.: Discussion of paper by Finney, J. M. T.: The relation of dilatation of the duodenum to gastric disturbance. Bull. Johns Hopkins Hosp. *17:*37 (Jan.) 1906.
7. Barnes, J. P.: Trocar decompression in acute small bowel obstruction. Surgery *37:*542–548 (Apr.) 1955.
8. Barnett, W. O., and Wall., L.: Megaduodenum resulting from absence of parasympathetic ganglion cells in Auerbach's plexus; review of literature and report of case. Ann. Surg. *141:*527–535 (Apr.) 1955.
9. Baron A.: Defect in broad ligament and its association with intestinal strangulation. Brit. J. Surg. *36:*91–94 (July) 1948.
10. Barry, H. C.: Fibrous stricture of small intestine following strangulated hernia. Brit. J. Surg. *30:*64–69 (July) 1942.
11. Becker, W. F.: Acute adhesive ileus; study of 412 cases with particular reference to abuse of tube decompression in treatment. Surg. Gynec. & Obst. *95:*472–476 (Oct.) 1952.
12. Bellis, C. J. and Wangensteen, O. H.: Venous circulatory changes in the abdomen and lower extremities attending intestinal distention. Proc. Soc. Exper. Biol. & Med. *41:*490–498 (June) 1939.
13. Berry, R. E.: Obstruction of the small bowel: an evaluation of pathology and treatment. Ann. Surg. *154:* Suppl. 102–111 (Dec.) 1961.

14. Bilgutay, A. M., Wingrove, R., Griffen, W. O., et al.: Gastro-intestinal pacing: a new concept in the treatment of ileus. Ann. Surg. *158:*338–348 (Sept.) 1963.
15. Bland, J. H.: Clinical Metabolism of Body Water and Electrolytes. Philadelphia, W. B. Saunders Co., 1963.
16. Bloodgood, J. C.: Acute dilatation of stomach—gastromesenteric ileus. Ann. Surg. *46:*736–762 (Nov.) 1907.
17. Bollinger, J. A., and Fowler, E. F.: Results of treatment of acute small bowel obstruction; clinical study of 205 consecutive cases. Arch. Surg. *66:*888–904 (June) 1953.
18. Bowles, H. E.: Hernia through broad ligament. Surgery *5:*382–388 (Mar.) 1939.
19. Boys, F.: Prophylaxis of peritoneal adhesions; review of literature. Surgery *11:*118–168 (Jan.) 1942.
20. Brayton, D., and Norris, W. J.: Intussusception in adults. Am. J. Surg. *88:*32–43 (July) 1954.
21. Brown, R. B., and Ross, D.: Congenital abnormalities of intestinal rotation and mesenteric attachment—cause of intestinal obstruction in adult. Ann. Surg. *134:*88–98 (July) 1951.
22. Bryant, L. R.: An evaluation of the effect of fibrinolysin on intraperitoneal adhesion formation. Am. J. Surg. *106:*892–897 (Dec.) 1963.
23. Cantor, M. O.: New simplified intestinal decompression tube. Am. J. Surg. *72:*137–142 (July) 1946.
24. Cantor, M. O., and Reynolds, R. P.: Gastro-intestinal Obstruction. Baltimore, The Williams & Wilkins Co., 1957.
25. Carp, L.: Foreign bodies in intestine. Ann. Surg. *85:*575–591 (Apr.) 1927.
26. Cattell, R. B., and Warren, K. W.: Surgery of the Pancreas. Philadelphia, W. B. Saunders Co., 1953.
27. Cohn, I., Jr.: Strangulation Obstruction. Springfield, Ill., Charles C Thomas, 1961.
28. Cohn, I., Jr.: The toxic factor in closed loop obstruction. Am. J. Surg. *104:*482–489 (Sept.) 1962.
29. Colcock, B. P., and Lamphier, T. A.: Endometriosis of large and small intestine. Surgery *28:*997–1004 (Dec.) 1950.
30. Cole, W. H., and Roberts, S.: Intestinal obstruction in adults. Am. Surgeon *28:*133–140 (Mar.) 1962.
31. Coletti, L., and Bossart, P. A.: Intestinal obstruction during the early postoperative period. Arch Surg. *88:*774–778 (May) 1964.
32. Coletti, L., Edmunds, R., Togut, A. J., et al.: Mechanical small bowel obstruction. Am. J. Surg. *104:*370–375 (Sept.) 1962.
33. Connolly, J. E., and Smith, J. W.: The prevention and treatment of intestinal adhesions. Internat. Abstr. Surg. *110:*417–431 (May) 1960; *in* Surg. Gynec. & Obst. *110* (May) 1960.
34. Dean, D. L., Ellis, F. H., Jr., and Sauer, W. G.: Intussusception in adults. Arch. Surg. *73:*6–11 (July) 1956.
35. DeBakey, M., and Ochsner, A.: Bezoars and concretions; comprehensive review of literature with analysis of 303 collected cases and presentation of 8 additional cases. Surgery *4:*934–963 (Dec.) 1938.
36. Dennis, C., and Varco, R. L.: Femoral hernia with gangrenous bowel. Surgery *22:*312–323 (Aug.) 1947.
37. Derblom, H., Johansson, H., and Nylander, G.: Small intestinal absorption and gastric secretion of iodide in total small bowel obstruction in the rat. Surgery *54:*771–783 (Nov.) 1963.
38. Donhauser, J. L., and Kelly, E. C.: Intussusception in adult. Am. J. Surg. *79:*673–677 (May) 1950.
39. Faber, K. I.: Perniciøs anaemia som følge af tarmlidelse. Hospitalstid. *4:*601–615, 1895.
40. Frimann-Dahl, J.: Postoperative Röntgenuntersuchungen; Diaphragmabewegungen und der postoperative Venenstrom; postoperative Lungenembolien. Acta chir. scandinav. (Supp. 36) *76:*1–168, 1935.
41. Gamble, J. L.: Chemical Anatomy, Physiology and Pathology of Extracellular Fluids: A Lecture Syllabus. Ed. 6. Dept. of Pediatrics, Harvard Med. School. Cambridge, Mass., Harvard University Press, 1954.
42. Gendel, S., and Fine, J.: Effect of acute intestinal obstruction on blood and plasma volumes. Ann. Surg. *110:*25–37 (July) 1939.

43. Gibson, J. M., Jr.: Gallstone ileus. Arch. Surg. *88*:297–298 (Feb.) 1964.
44. Girdwood, R. H.: Disorders of alimentary tract and their nutritional effects; absorption of vitamins in disorders of alimentary tract. Proc. Nutrition Soc. *14*:41–50, 1955.
45. Goin, L. S., and Wilk, S. P.: Intermittent arteriomesenteric occlusion of duodenum. Radiology *67*:729–736 (Nov.) 1956.
46. Harkins, H. N.: Intussusception due to invaginated Meckel's diverticulum; report of 2 cases with study of 160 cases collected from literature. Ann. Surg. *98*:1070–1095 (Dec.) 1933.
47. Harrison, B. F., Jr., and Cheek, J. H.: Intersigmoid hernia; review of literature and report of additional case. Texas J. Med. *47*:776–779 (Nov.) 1951.
48. Hibbard, J. S., and Wangensteen, O. H.: Character of gaseous distention in mechanical obstruction of small intestine. Proc. Soc. Exper. Biol. & Med. *31*:1063–1066 (June) 1934.
49. Hill, F. C., O'Loughlin, B. J., and Stoner, M.: Peritoneal aspiration in diagnosis of strangulated bowel. Surg. Gynec. & Obst. *74*:121–123 (Jan.) 1942.
50. Kantor, J. L.: Common anomalies of duodenum and colon: their practical significance; result of 8 years' combined clinical and roentgen study. J.A.M.A. *97*:1785–1790 (Dec. 12) 1931.
51. Keynes, W. M.: Richter's hernia. Surg. Gynec. & Obst. *103*:496–500 (Oct.) 1956.
52. Koontz, A. R.: Hernia. New York, Appleton-Century-Crofts, 1963.
53. Kostlivy, S.: Ueber den anatomischen und funktionellen Anteil bei der Entstehung der chronischen relativen infrapapillaren Duodenalstenose. Mitt. a. d. Grenzgeb. d. Med. u. Chir. *42*:282–294, 1931.
54. Langley, G. F.: Strangulated internal hernia: report of cases of strangulation in fossa iliaco-subfascialis and through foramen of Winslow. Brit. J. Surg. *23*:119–127 (July) 1935.
55. Larson, D. L., Karzel, R., and Cameron, H.: Intestinal intubation with the aid of a magnetic tube. Surg. Gynec. & Obst. *115*:503–504 (Oct.) 1962.
56. Laufman, H., and Nora, P. F.: Physiological problems underlying intestinal strangulation obstruction. S. Clin. North America *42*:219–229 (Feb.) 1962.
57. Law, D. H., and Ten Eyck, E. A.: Familial megaduodenum and megacystis. Am. J. Med. *33*:911–922 (Dec.) 1962.
58. Leonard, A. S., Nicoloff, D. M., Griffen, W. O., Jr., et al.: Long coiled spring tube for operative intestinal decompression. Am. J. Surg. *104*:427–432 (Sept.) 1962.
59. Levey, S., Abbott, W. E., Krieger, H., et al.: Metabolic alterations in surgical patients; studies involving iron and magnesium metabolism in patients with gastrointestinal drainage. J. Lab. & Clin. Med. *47*:437–443 (Mar.) 1956.
60. Levin, A. L.: New gastroduodenal catheter. J.A.M.A. *76*:1007 (Apr. 9) 1921.
61. Little, W. D., Zerfas, L. G., and Trusler, H. M.: Chronic obstruction of the small bowel. The result of two entero-enterostomies and apparently the cause of pernicious anemia. J.A.M.A. *93*:1290–1291 (Oct. 26) 1929.
62. MacQuiddy, E. L., and Tollman, J. P.: Observations on absorbable powder to replace talc. Surgery *23*:786–793 (May) 1948.
63. Major, J. W., Ottenheimer, E. J., and Whalen, W. A., Jr.: Duodenal obstruction at the ligament of Treitz. Report of a case treated by a plastic procedure. New England J. Med. *262*:443–445 (Mar. 3) 1960.
64. Martin, F.: Intestinal obstruction due to gallstones; with report of three successful cases. Ann. Surg. *55*:725–743 (May) 1912.
65. Martorell, R.: Jejunal obstructions. Am. J. Surg. *104*:433–438 (Sept.) 1962.
66. Matheson, N. A., and Dudley, H. A.: Enterotomy and decompression for intestinal distension. Lancet *1*:695–696 (Mar. 30) 1963.
67. May, S. C., and Brintnall, E. S.: Strangulated transmesenteric hernia in erythroblastotic newborn (report of case treated by resection and anastomosis with survival). Surgery *33*:312–314 (Feb.) 1953.
68. McCune, W. S.: Tube jejunostomy in treatment of recurrent small bowel obstruction. Am. J. Surg. *27*:778–783 (Nov.) 1961.
69. McKittrick, L. S., and Sarris, S. P.: Acute mechanical obstruction of small bowel; diagnosis and treatment. New England J. Med. *222*:611–622 (Apr. 11) 1940.
70. McLaughlin, C. W., Jr., and Raines, M.: Obstruction of alimentary tract from gallstones. Am. J. Surg. *81*:424–430 (Apr.) 1951.

71. McVay, C. B., and Anson, B. J.: Fundamental error in current methods of inguinal herniorrhaphy. Surg. Gynec. & Obst. *74:*746–750 (Mar.) 1942.
72. Mikal, S. J.: Fluid and electrolyte abnormalities in small bowel obstruction. Am. J. Proctol. *13:*243–248 (Aug.) 1962.
73. Miller, T. G., and Abbott, W. O.: Intestinal intubation: practical technique. Am. J. M. Sc. *187:*595–599 (May) 1934.
74. Moore, T. C.: Transmesenteric hernia in infancy; with a note on operative intestinal decompression in infancy. Surgery *41:*438–443 (Mar.) 1957.
75. Moore, T. C., and Baker, W. H.: Operative and radiologic relief of gallstone intestinal obstruction. Surg. Gynec. & Obst. *116:*189–195 (Feb.) 1963.
76. Moyer, C. A.: Fluid Balance: A Clinical Manual. Chicago, Year Book Medical Publishers, 1952.
77. Nell, W.: Ein beitrag zur Atiologie des "Echten" Megaduodenums. Beitr. klin. Chir. *157:*401–413, 1933.
78. Nemir, P., Jr., Hawthorne, H. R., Cohn, I., Jr., et al.: Cause of death in strangulation obstruction: experimental study; clinical course, chemical, bacteriologic and spectrophotometric studies. Ann. Surg. *130:*857–873 (Nov.) 1949.
79. Nemir, P., Jr., Hawthorne, H. R., Cohn, I., Jr., et al.: Cause of death in strangulation obstruction: experimental study; lethal action of peritoneal fluid. Ann. Surg. *130:*874–880 (Nov.) 1949.
80. Noble, T. B., Jr.: Plication of small intestine as prophylaxis against adhesions. Am. J. Surg. *35:*41–44 (Jan.) 1937.
81. Norberg, P. B.: Food as a cause of intestinal obstruction. Am. J. Surg. *104:*444–447 (Sept.) 1962.
82. Nugent, F. W., Braasch, J. W., and Epstein, H.: Diagnosis and surgical treatment of arteriomesenteric obstruction of the duodenum. J.A.M.A. *196:*1091–1093 (June 20) 1966.
83. Ostrum, B. J., and Heinz, E. R.: Small bowel obstruction versus adynamic ileus. A study using a water soluble oral contrast material. Am. J. Roentgenol. *89:*734–739 (Apr.) 1963.
84. Petit, L. A.: De L'Etranglement du Duodenum au Niveau de la Racine du Mesentere. Paris, G. Steinheil, 1900.
85. Poth, E. J.: Plication in the surgical treatment of chronic recurrent intestinal obstruction. Am. J. Surg. *104:*413–418 (Sept.) 1962.
86. Quan, S. H., and Stearns, M. W., Jr.: Early postoperative intestinal obstruction and postoperative intestinal ileus. Dis. Colon & Rectum *4:*307–318 (Sept.-Oct.) 1961.
87. Quast, D. C., Beall, A. C., Jr., and DeBakey, M. E.: Clinical evaluation of the gastrointestinal pacer. Surg. Gynec. & Obst. *120:*35–37 (Jan.) 1965.
88. Rabinovitch, J., Pines, B., and Felton, M.: Superior mesenteric artery syndrome. J.A.M.A. *179:*257–263 (Jan. 27) 1962.
89. Richter, A. G.: Hernia. Goettingen, J. C. Dieterich, 1785, p. 597.
90. Ripstein, C. B., and Miller, G. G.: Volvulus of small intestine. Surgery *27:*506–511 (Apr.) 1950.
91. Roberts, K. E., Vanamee, P., and Poppell, J. W.: Electrolyte Changes in Surgery. Springfield, Ill., Charles C Thomas, 1958.
92. Saltzstein, E. C., Marshall, W. J., and Freeark, R. J.: Gangrenous intestinal obstruction. Surg. Gynec. & Obst. *114:*694–700 (June) 1962.
93. Sherwin, B., and Rockey, E. E.: Duodenal obstruction caused by chronic pyelonephritis and hydronephrosis. New York J. Med. *46:*414–416 (Feb. 15) 1946.
94. Silen, W., Hein, M. F., and Goldman, L.: Strangulation obstruction of the small intestine. Arch. Surg. *85:*121–129 (July) 1962.
95. Smith, G. A.: Study of intestinal intubation using flexible stylet with controllable tip. Surgery *32:*17–30 (July) 1952.
96. Smith, G. A., Perry, J. F., Jr., and Yonehiro, E. G.: Mechanical intestinal obstructions; study of 1,252 cases. Surg. Gynec. & Obst. *100:*651–660 (June) 1955.
97. Strong, E. K.: Mechanics of arteriomesenteric duodenal obstruction and direct surgical attack upon etiology. Ann. Surg. *148:*725–730 (Nov.) 1958.
98. Tendler, M. J., and Ciuti, A.: Surgery of annular pancreas; summary of 60 patients operated upon. Surgery *38:*298–310 (Aug.) 1955.
99. Turner, M. D., Grogan, J. B., and Truett, G. W.: A study of the lethal mechanism in

experimental closed loop strangulated obstruction of the small intestine. Am. J. Surg. *102*:560–568 (Oct.) 1961.
100. Turner, R. H.: Pellagra associated with organic disease of gastro-intestinal tract. Am. J. Trop. Med. *9*:129–137 (Mar.) 1929.
101. Tyson, W. T., Jr., and Keegan, J. M.: Duodenal obstruction due to compression by superior mesenteric root. J.A.M.A. *165*:1665–1668 (Nov. 30) 1957.
102. U. S. Bureau of Census, Statistical Abstracts of the United States: 1963. Ed. 84. Washington, D.C., 1963, p. 65.
103. Venner, B.: Hernia through foramen of Winslow. M. J. Australia *2*:678 (Nov. 5) 1949.
104. Vest, B.: Roentgenographic diagnosis of strangulating closed-loop obstruction of the small intestine. Surg. Gynec. & Obst. *115*:561–567 (Nov.) 1962.
105. Vest, B., and Margulis, A. R.: The roentgen diagnosis of postoperative ileus-obstruction. Surg. Gynec. & Obst. *115*:421–427 (Oct.) 1962.
106. Wang, C. A., and Welch, C. E.: Anomalies of intestinal rotation in adolescents and adults. Surgery *54*:839–855 (Dec.) 1963.
107. Wangensteen, O. H.: The early diagnosis of acute intestinal obstruction with comments on pathology and treatment; with report of successful decompression of three cases of mechanical bowel obstruction by nasal catheter suction siphonage. West. J. Surg. *40*:1–17 (Jan.) 1932.
108. Wangensteen, O. H., and Rea, C. E.: The distention factor in simple intestinal obstruction: An experimental study with exclusion of swallowed air by cervical esophagostomy. Surgery *5*:327–339 (Mar.) 1939.
109. Welch, C. E.: Intestinal Obstruction. Chicago, Year Book Publishers, Inc., 1958.
110. Westerman, C. W. J.: Über die anwendung des Dauermagenhebers bei der Nachbehandlung schwerer Peritonitisfalle. Zentralbl. Chir. *37*:356–357 (Mar. 5) 1910.
111. White, R. R.: Prevention of recurrent small bowel obstruction due to adhesions. Ann. Surg. *143*:714–719 (May) 1956.
112. Wilson, N. D.: Complications of the Noble procedure. Am. J. Surg. *108*:264–269 (Aug.) 1964.
113. Yull, A. B., Abrams, J. S., and Davis, J. H.: The peritoneal fluid in strangulation obstruction. The role of the red blood cell and E. coli bacteria in producing toxicity. J. Surg. Research *2*:223–232 (July) 1962.

Chapter Four

TUMORS

In common with other portions of the alimentary tract, the small intestine gives rise to a large number of new growths. In fact, almost all the cells that histologically make up the small bowel have representation in the benign and malignant types of small intestinal neoplasms. Thus, a compilation of such tumors as reported in the literature, is extensive and includes 35 varieties (Table 4–1). In clinical consideration of such tumors,

Table 4–1. Compilation of Small Intestinal Neoplasms Showing Frequency at One Institution*

BENIGN	358	MALIGNANT	185
Leiomyoma	120	Adenocarcinoma	93
Lipoma	67	Leiomyosarcoma	36
Adenomatous polyp	67	Lymphosarcoma	26
Hemangioma	57	Reticulum cell sarcoma	15
Lymphangioma	16	Hodgkin's sarcoma	10
Fibroma	11	Hemangioendothelioma	3
Brunner's gland adenoma	6	Giant follicular lymphoma	1
Neurofibroma	4	Lymphangioendothelioma	1
Gastric mucosa adenoma	2		
Adenomyoma	2	CARCINOIDS	163
Adenofibroma	1		
Lipoleiomyoma	1	OTHER LESIONS FROM WORLD'S LITERATURE (RARE)	
Cystadenoma	1	Fibrosarcoma; Teratoma	
Endometrioma	1	Lymphocytoma; Hamartoma	
Ganglioneuroma	1	Plasmocytoma; Reticulofibromatosis	
Myxoma	1	Osteofibroma; Hemangiopericytoma	
		Osteoma; Aberrant pancreatic tissue	

*Autopsy and surgical cases from 1938 through 1957 at the Mayo Clinic. Adapted from Moertel, C. G., et al.: Cancer *14*:903 (Sept.-Oct.) 1961.

it is helpful to keep in mind that there are four major groups—carcinomas, sarcomas, carcinoids, and the benign tumors.

The total number of small bowel neoplasms reported in the literature is relatively small. Up to 1960, Rochlin and Longmire[54] found 650 reported cases of malignant tumors. In a survey of the world literature through December of 1954, River et al.[53] compiled 1399 cases of benign small bowel tumors. As a further index of their infrequency, Shallow et al.[56] have found that small bowel malignancies occurred in from 0.03 to 1.5 percent of autopsy series. The earlier literature indicated that there were 100 carcinomas of the stomach and colon found for every case of small bowel carcinoma discovered.[32] Comparatively speaking, benign tumors are found as frequently as the malignant varieties except in autopsy series where they outnumber malignant tumors.[1, 4] Among the malignant tumors, carcinomas, sarcomas, and carcinoid tumors are found in a ratio of 3:2:1.[27, 54]

Neoplasms of the small bowel occur in later life, most commonly in the fifth to seventh decades.[5] The sex distribution is about equal.[4, 5] Rankin and Newell,[48] Cameron,[7] and Mayo,[31] however, found the ratio of males to females to be 2:1.

DIAGNOSIS

SYMPTOMS AND SIGNS

The most prominent symptoms associated with tumors of the small bowel are pain, nausea, and vomiting. The clinical courses of patients with small bowel tumors are predictable from their forms of growth (Fig. 4–1). They may be intraluminal and form large bulky growths. Such tumors often lead to intussusception and obstruction (Fig. 4–2). They may infiltrate the wall of the bowel and constrict its lumen (Fig. 4–3). A third type expands under the serosa, forming a pedunculated tumor emerging from the surface, which may attain a large size and be associated with volvulus.

Because of mucosal or submucosal involvement, a less common presenting symptom is hemorrhage. Melena of either tarry or grossly bloody stools may be prominent. The bleeding may be occult with resultant severe anemia. Bleeding is more common from vascular tumors and the myomas. Thus, benign hemangiomas, malignant hemangioendotheliomas, leiomyomas, and leiomyosarcomas make up a large proportion of the tumors in cases with hemorrhage.

Botsford et al.[5] reported 34 instances of benign and malignant tumors causing intestinal obstruction, 9 causing bleeding, and 7 causing abdominal pain without obstruction. Strohl and Diffenbaugh[64] reported weight loss in

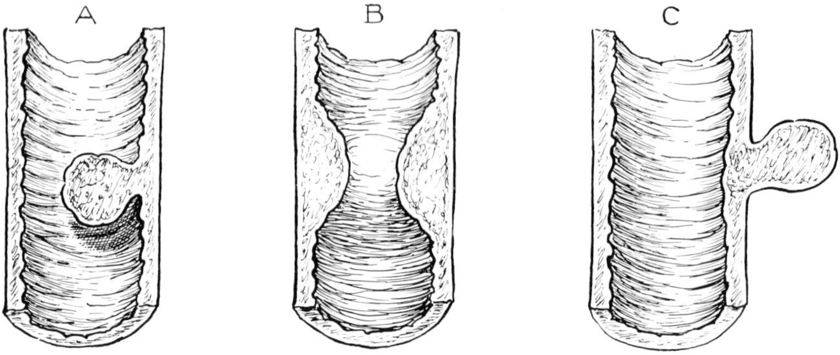

Figure 4–1. Forms of growth of small intestinal neoplasms (intraluminal polypoid, intramural, and serosal).

82 percent, obstruction in 75 percent, nausea and vomiting in 64 percent, pain in 57 percent, and diarrhea in 25 percent. The physical findings were anemia in 64 percent, abdominal distention in 57 percent, and palpable mass in 43 percent. Rochlin and Longmire[54] emphasized the symptom complex in which tenesmus and diarrhea with mucus was prominent. Weibel et al.[69] confirmed these reports and found a palpable mass in 29 percent of malignant tumors. Obstruction of the biliary tract is common with malignant tumors of the second portion of the duodenum.

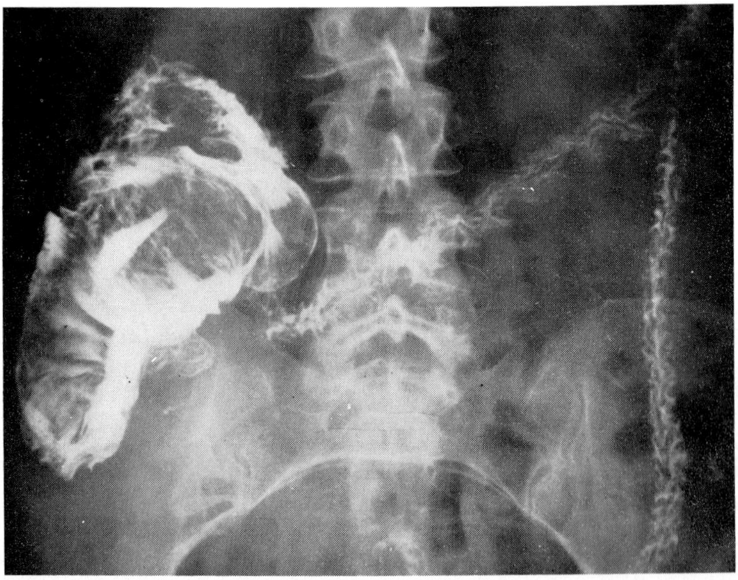

Figure 4–2. Barium enema showing ileocecal intussusception due to ileal neoplasm.

RADIOLOGIC DIAGNOSIS

The accuracy of roentgenographic diagnosis of small bowel tumors is variable. Until recently, fractional barium examination of the small bowel has not been useful in visualizing early small tumors. The fact that tumors are large by the time the diagnostician and later the radiologist are consulted explains the high success rate of 90 percent reported by Weber and Kirklin[68] and the high rate of Golden and Morales.[18] Conversely, Keats and Sakai[26] reported a success rate for visualization of 59 percent. It should be noted that this latter series included autopsy cases of benign as well as malignant tumors. A small benign tumor of the kind frequently discovered at autopsy must of necessity be more difficult to visualize radiographically than a large symptomatic malignant tumor.

The conventional technique for radiographic visualization of the small bowel is the so-called fractional visualization carried out at half hour intervals after barium ingestion. With this method, the stigmata of small bowel tumors,[26] annular constriction, filling defects, obstruction, mucosal distortion, ulceration, extrinsic pressure deformity, and intussusception may be obscured by overlapping of loops and retained barium in the stomach.[24] One must keep in mind that unexplained delay or dilatation is a possible sign of tumor, probably a malignant tumor. The addition of fluoroscopy with palpation to separate loops is an important technique. Above all, to improve the results of small bowel visualization, it must be realized that careful studies bear diagnostic fruit. In the future the possible use of cineradiography with "playback" seems to promise improvement in diagnostic accuracy.

Another method described by Schatzki[55] depends on distention of the entire small bowel by administration of barium through a tube in the jejunum. This technique has not been widely accepted.

MALIGNANT SMALL INTESTINAL TUMORS

ADENOCARCINOMA

Adenocarcinoma of the small bowel is the most common malignant tumor of the small intestine (Fig. 4–3).[54] It is more common in the duodenum, with a decreasing incidence in the more distal portions of the small intestine.[4] Within the duodenum, its location can be conveniently designated as a suprapapillary, papillary, or infrapapillary position. This division is natural as the presenting symptom of the papillary location commonly is jaundice (Fig. 4–4). Carcinomas of all portions of the duodenum have a tendency to bleed. Adenocarcinoma of the jejunum or ileum is frequently heralded by the pain of partial obstruction.

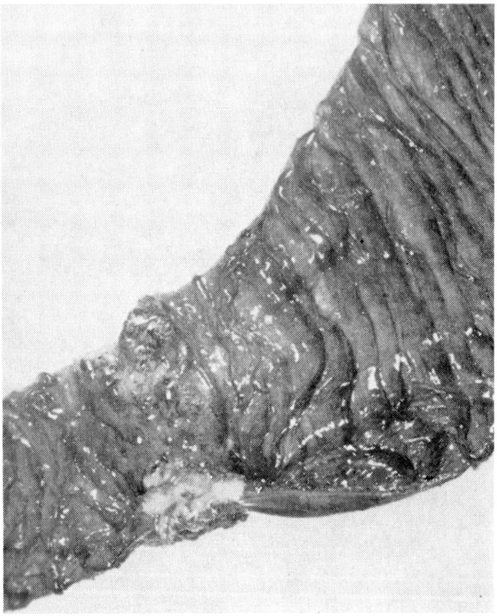

Figure 4–3. Adenocarcinoma of jejunum causing partial obstruction as a result of constriction of the intramural lesion.

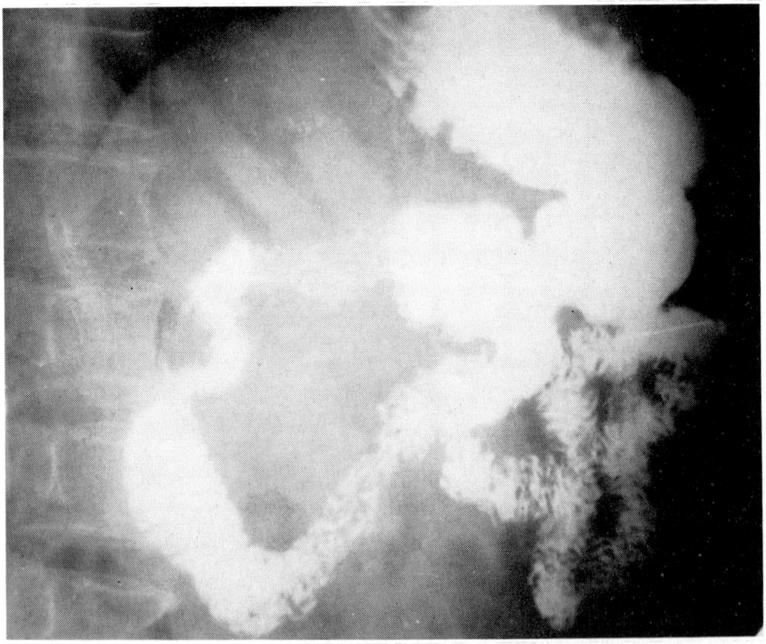

Figure 4–4. Adenocarcinoma of the papillary portion of the duodenum.

The treatment of adenocarcinoma of the small intestine is resection, including in the removed specimen as much of the mesentery as possible. Frequently this procedure is not practicable for two reasons. First, about half of all adenocarcinomas have metastasized widely to the mesenteric and periaortic lymph nodes, and the resection is palliative. Second, the location of duodenal adenocarcinoma in close proximity to the pancreas and the lack of mesentery to the duodenum do not permit a wide en bloc resection. For these reasons, cure or five-year survival does not occur frequently. A five-year survival rate of 20 percent as reported by Rochlin and Longmire[54] is comparatively favorable, as is the five-year survival rate of 39 percent in a series of duodenal carcinomas reported by Cattell et al.[8]

SARCOMA

Clinically, sarcomas as a group do not differ appreciably from carcinomas. Sarcomas are more common in the ileum than proximally in the duodenum and jejunum. They tend to grow external to the bowel and, therefore, are more likely to be palpable and less likely to produce signs and symptoms of intestinal obstruction.

LYMPHOMA

The types of sarcoma are listed in Table 4–1. The most common is the lymphoma, the classification of which is found in Table 4–2. The relationship of the systemic disease to the form localized in the intestine is not clear. This discussion is limited to those lymphomas apparently localized in the small intestine or its environs—which accounted for 11 percent of 618 cases of lymphoma in all locations reviewed by Gall and Mallory.[13]

Since pathologists do not agree on the proper classification of lymphomas of the small intestine, and since the condition is rare, it is difficult to arrive at definite conclusions concerning them. Apparently they are more common in the lower portion of the small bowel and in males, are occasionally multiple, and according to some authors are prone to perforation with or

Table 4–2. Meissner's Classification of Lymphomas*

Lymphoma, unclassified
Lymphosarcoma
Lymphocytoma
Reticulum cell sarcoma
Macrofollicular lymphoma
Hodgkin's disease

*Adapted from Warren, K. W., and Littlefield, J. B.: S. Clin. North America *35:*737 (June) 1955.

without radiation treatment.[4] They occasionally are associated with malabsorption and pneumatosis intestinalis.[70]

The treatment is usually resection with removal of as much of the mesentery as possible and a wide free margin of intestine. Frozen section examination of the margins of the resected specimen is advisable as the submucosal spread of lymphomas of the stomach is notorious. The results of surgery as summarized by Bernstein and Chey[4] indicate that the long-term survival varies from 10 to 40 percent. Unremoved disease is not a harbinger of early death, because patients with appreciable longevity are recorded under these circumstances. The place of radiation therapy is not certain although Warren and Littlefield[66] reported long-term survival in two cases after gastroenterostomy and radiation for lymphoma of the duodenum. In fact, they suggested that resection for lymphoma of the duodenum is not indicated.

LEIOMYOSARCOMA

Prominent among other sarcomas are the leiomyosarcomas. Starr and Dockerty[62] reviewed this subject comprehensively, and pointed out that these tumors differ clinically from other malignant tumors by a high incidence of bleeding, the large size they frequently attain, and their compatibility with long life despite the presence of metastasis. In the series reported by Starr and Dockerty, approximately 50 percent of patients with leiomyosarcoma survived for five years.

OTHER MALIGNANT TUMORS

Malignant vascular tumors are described elsewhere in this chapter and in the chapter on vascular malformations. For a more extensive consideration of other sarcomas, one of the comprehensive reviews on the subject should be consulted.[54]

CARCINOID TUMORS

GENERAL CONSIDERATIONS

The subject of carcinoid tumors of the small intestine has evoked considerable interest in the last decade among surgeons, internists, and pathologists because of the wide range of growth potential shown by these lesions and an unusual syndrome associated with them. Whereas almost all appendiceal carcinoids lack the ability for metastatic spread,[29] some ileal carcinoids have a high growth potential. As one author noted, the number of published articles on carcinoid tumors is greater than the number of reported tumors.[36]

First described clearly by Lubarsch in 1888[28] and again by Ŕansom[49] in 1890, the malignancy of carcinoid tumors was first recognized by Aschoff[2] in 1911 and the origin of carcinoid tumors ascribed by Masson[30] in the 1920's to the Kultschitzky cell in the crypts of Lieberkühn. Masson's identification of carcinoid cells with Kultschitzky's cells is based on a similarity in staining reaction of certain globules in the cytoplasm to a silver stain. That this staining reaction is not specific and that carcinoids of the bronchus (some of which are functioning) do not fit this association have been overlooked since Masson's convincing arguments. In addition, Masson suggested that carcinoid tumors were endocrine in nature. Confirmatory observations in this regard did not come until 25 years later with the publications of Isler and Hedinger[22] and of Thorson et al.[65]

Carcinoid tumors can occur at any location in the gastrointestinal tract from the gastric cardia to the anus and thus involve structures developed from the primitive entoderm.[29] A few have been reported in teratomas, an understandable aberration.[45] Another has been found in a Meckel's diverticulum and was associated with hepatic metastasis and the carcinoid syndrome.[60]

The location of gastrointestinal carcinoids in a large series is shown in Table 4–3. The majority (45.9 percent) were primary in the appendix; the next structures most frequently involved were the ileum (27.9 percent) and the rectum (16.7 percent).

These tumors are small, the majority being less than 1.5 cm. in diameter.[36] Characteristically, they are located in the mucosal layers and are yellowish or white (Fig. 4–5). The size of the lesion seems important, since few lesions (2 percent) less than 1 cm. in diameter showed metastasis. They are frequently multiple (29 percent) and, in addition, often are associated with other primary malignant neoplasms (17 to 53 percent).

Table 4–3. Location of Gastrointestinal Carcinoids*

SITE	NUMBER OF CASES	DISTRIBUTION (*percent*)
Stomach	83	2.8
Gallbladder	8	0.3
Duodenum	43	1.5
Jejunum	49	1.7
Ileum	813	27.9
Meckel's diverticulum	33	1.1
Appendix	1340	45.9
Colon	61	2.1
Rectum	486	16.7
Total	2916	100.0

*Adapted from Postlethwait, R. W.: Postgrad. Med. *40*:447 (Oct.) 1966.

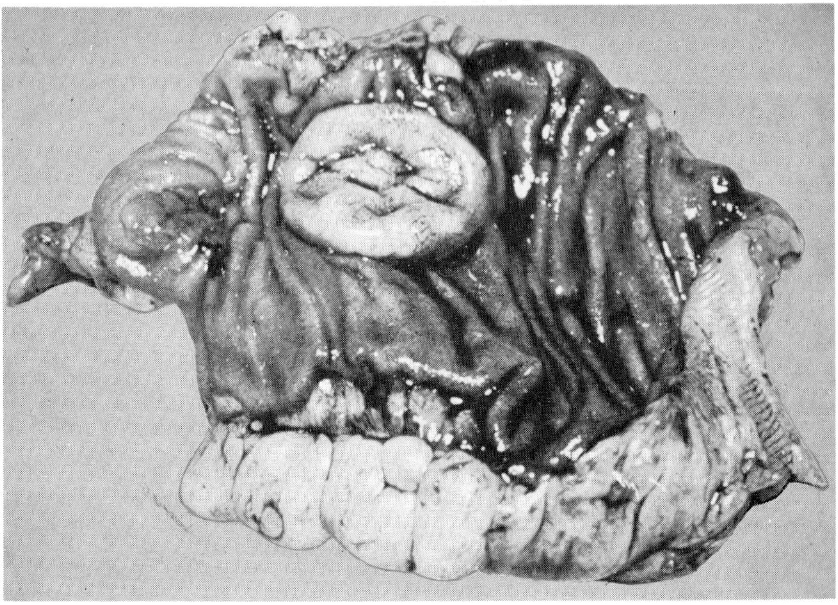

Figure 4–5. Carcinoid tumor of ileum. This patient had massive metastatic disease in the liver and the carcinoid syndrome.

Because of an intense fibroblastic reaction surrounding metastatic disease in the mesenteric nodes, buckling of the bowel results, with subsequent obstruction of the lumen. Metastasis to the lymph nodes and liver, with occasional peritoneal seeding, and spread to the ovary are the usual extent of these metastatic lesions. Extraabdominal spread is unusual. Bone is the commonest extraabdominal site of metastasis.

In planning the treatment of a patient with a small intestinal carcinoid it is important to know the life history of this tumor. Data regarding metastatic habits of the tumor have been published by MacDonald (Table 4–4).[29] It must be remembered that a somewhat higher incidence of all types of invasiveness would be encountered in any purely clinical series since these

Table 4–4. Invasiveness of Carcinoid Tumors of Small Intestine*

LOCATION	TOTAL CASES	NONINVASIVE	INVASIVE *Muscle*	*Nodes*	DISTANT
Duodenum	8	5	2	0	1
Jejunum	17	7	4	4	2
Ileum	73	26	24	15	8
Meckel's diverticulum	2	2	0	0	0
Total	100	40	30	19	11

*Adapted from MacDonald, R. A.: Am. J. Med. *21*:869 (Dec.) 1956.

Table 4-5. Duration of Life From Onset of Symptoms of Carcinoid Tumor to Death From Metastases*

DURATION OF LIFE (*years*)	NO. OF CASES	PERCENT
1	2	7
1–4	11	39
5–9	8	29
10–14	1	4
15–19	3	11
20–24	3	11

*Adapted from Moertel, C. G., et al.: Cancer *14*:911 (Sept.-Oct.) 1961.

tumors cause symptoms (obstruction usually) late in their clinical course. The MacDonald series is derived in part (28 percent) from autopsy material in which the tumor was an incidental finding. In any case, 23 of 73 ileal carcinoids (32 percent) showed metastasis to nodes or distant sites. The comparable figure for the jejunum was 35 percent.

The life expectancy of patients with metastatic carcinoid tumors has been studied by Moertel et al.[36] and shown to average 8.1 years (Table 4-5). Three of his patients lived 20 to 24 years after the onset of symptoms. Thus, life expectancy even with metastasis is completely variable and unpredictable.

The treatment of carcinoid tumors of the small intestine is resection of the primary lesion en bloc with its mesenteric lymphogenous drainage area. Even in patients with hepatic, peritoneal, or irremovable nodal metastatic disease, resection of as much of the bulk of the tumor as is compatible with safety is desirable. A case in point is described by Moertel et al.[36] This patient lived in comfort for 14 years with known nonresectable tumor in the mesenteric and aortic nodes, only to die of unrelated disease. In a series[36] of 17 patients with resectable metastatic tumors, 12 (71 percent) survived five years or more after operation. Of 22 patients with nonresectable metastases, 6 patients (27 percent) survived for five years. Indeed, a malignant neoplasm in slow motion is an apt description for this unusual tumor.

CARCINOID SYNDROME

The presence of a bizarre series of signs and symptoms associated with metastatic carcinoid tumors has been well documented.[65] Characteristically, the symptoms include a peculiar dark red or purplish flush intermittently involving the trunk and, in particular, the face. The flush usually starts abruptly and may be precipitated by food, alcohol, or emotional stress. Ordinarily its duration is brief, but it may last several hours. Another common symptom of the syndrome is diarrhea. Occasionally, asthma, tachycardia, arthralgia, and pellagra-like skin changes are associated. At necropsy, subendothelial fibrosis of the pulmonic or tricuspid valve, or both, is seen, leading to pulmonic stenosis or tricuspid insufficiency. This syndrome can be disabling because of intractable diarrhea, frequent flushing, cardiac failure as a result of valvular changes, or any combination of these signs and symptoms.

The incidence of this syndrome is low. Up to 1956, MacDonald[29] found 53 acceptable cases. Moertel et al.[36] reported 14 additional cases in 1961 from the Mayo Clinic. Of 143 patients without metastasis reported by Moertel et al., none had symptoms of this syndrome; of 32 patients with nodal metastases, only 2 had the carcinoid syndrome. However, of 34 patients with hepatic metastasis, 12, or 35 percent, noted the symptoms of the carcinoid syndrome.

Speculation regarding the pathogenesis of the carcinoid syndrome has led to the following theory: carcinoid tissue, in particular metastatic disease in the liver and occasionally massive deposits in the mesentery, secretes a substance, serotonin (5-hydroxytryptamine).[10, 36] Ordinarily, 5-hydroxytryptamine is changed by a monamine oxidase in the liver to 5-hydroxyindoleacetic acid, a pharmacologically inactive substance. In some situations, however, blood returning to the heart with a high content of serotonin has bypassed the functioning liver tissue (from hepatic metastasis or ovarian teratomas containing carcinoid tissue), and serotonin reaches the heart and peripheral circulation in major concentrations. Thus, high concentrations of serotonin in the heart tissue and peripheral areas are thought to produce the syndrome.

In support of this theory are the following observations: serotonin has been extracted from carcinoid tumors; the metabolic end product of serotonin, 5-hydroxy-indoleacetic acid, is excreted in the urine of patients with the carcinoid syndrome in amounts up to 100 or 150 times normal, which allows confirmation of the clinical diagnosis;[57] approximately two thirds of the serotonin not bound to platelets in the blood is removed by a passage through the lungs, thus explaining the right-sided heart lesions;[17] the same workers pointed out the high content of monamine oxidase, a substance that is known to convert serotonin to 5-hydroxy-indoleacetic acid, in lung tissue; an interesting case of the carcinoid syndrome in a patient with a patent foramen ovale and involvement of both sides of the heart has been reported.[33]

Conversely, the serotonin content of tumors associated with the carcinoid syndrome varies widely;[10] injection of serotonin in varying amounts does not reproduce the syndrome;[43, 44] and the administration of serotonin antagonists or agents to block production of serotonin has not been particularly effective in ameliorating the syndrome.[11, 35, 42, 59]

Despite a lack of direct implication of serotonin in the production of the syndrome, it does seem likely that there is a close relationship between this chemical and the distressing symptoms of the syndrome.

The precise recognition of this syndrome is dependent on the demonstration of a higher than normal urinary excretion of the end product of serotonin metabolism in the urine, 5-hydroxy-indoleacetic acid. A simple quantitative test has been described by Sjoerdsma et al.[57] Bananas and certain medications must be excluded from the diet during the time the urine is collected, or a positive result is without meaning.

The treatment of patients afflicted with this syndrome is usually unsatisfactory. The use of agents that block serotonin synthesis or the use of serotonin antagonists often is ineffective.[11, 35, 58] On the other hand, large masses of functioning metastatic tissue have been removed successfully by partial hepatectomy,[9, 39, 61, 71] excision of large masses of involved mesenteric nodes,[36] or excision of an ovarian teratoma containing argentaffin cells.[45] Thus, if the major part of the functioning carcinoid metastatic tumor can be surgically excised, long-lasting relief of symptoms can usually be obtained.

5-Fluorouracil infusion of a liver containing metastatic carcinoid tumor with amelioration of the symptoms of the syndrome has been reported by Reed et al.[51] The catheter for infusion was introduced into the brachial artery and advanced into the hepatic artery by way of the descending aorta.

In the majority of successful cases, lowered urinary excretion of products of serotonin metabolism coincidental to the relief of symptoms has been documented.

In considering liver resection, it must be remembered that about 10 percent of patients with metastatic carcinoid disease are dead within one year or less of the onset of symptoms. Approximately 40 percent live only one to four years. It would not seem worth while, therefore, to subject the patient to liver resection with limited benefits if the life expectancy is only a year or so. If the tumor does not progress rapidly, and if the symptoms are severe, greater risks can be taken and massive liver resection seems indicated.

The type of anesthesia for surgical procedures on patients with the carcinoid syndrome is an important consideration. Sudden alteration of the blood pressure or a difficult induction period may be responsible for a large outpouring of serotonin into the general circulation. This sequence of events has been known to cause disaster. For this reason, Stone and Donnelly[63] advise the avoidance of spinal anesthesia and emphasize the importance of a gentle induction.

BENIGN SMALL INTESTINAL TUMORS

General Considerations

Benign neoplasms of the small intestine are of exceedingly great variety,[36, 51, 53] and their various forms encompass several fascinating groups of tumors (Table 4–1). In a monumental work published in 1956, River,

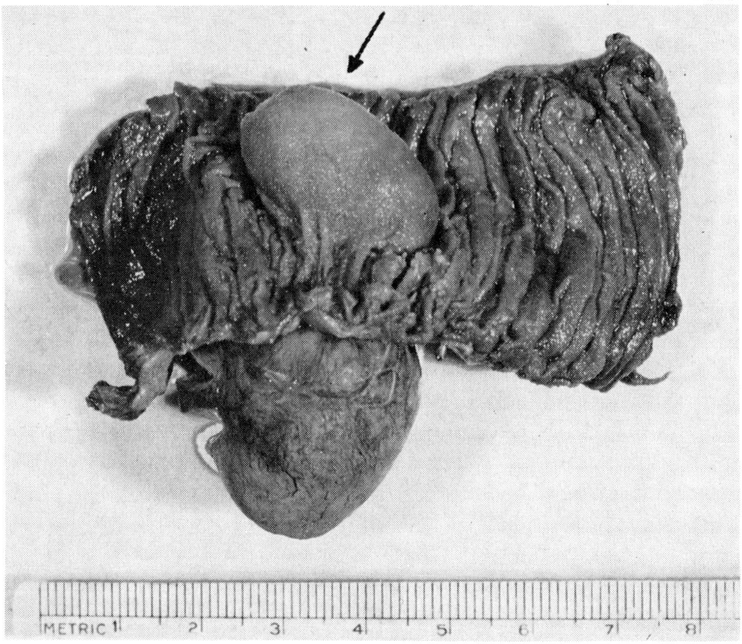

Figure 4–6. Leiomyoma of jejunum (arrow); note submucosal position. The second lesion is a diverticulum.

Silverstein, and Tope[53] collected and discussed 1399 cases of benign neoplasms of the small intestine compiled from the literature and from the files of the Cook County Hospital in Chicago. In addition, over 300 similar tumors from the Mayo Clinic were reviewed. Over 1000 references were listed.

The incidence of benign small bowel tumors is of the same order of magnitude as the malignant varieties. The symptomatology of benign tumors is also similar to that of malignant ones in that obstruction, with abdominal pain, nausea, and vomiting, is prevalent. Usually the obstruction is caused by an intussusception, of which the tumor is the leading point. Next in importance is hemorrhage, with melena and anemia. The hemorrhage may be massive and result in shock and death, or the bleeding may be occult and of long duration. This complication is most prominent with myomas and vascular tumors.[53] In the majority of cases, severe exsanguinating bleeding was the result of ulceration of the mucosa over submucosal growths (Fig. 4–6). Other complications that occur much less frequently include peritonitis, fistula formation, and malignant transformation.

ASSOCIATION WITH OTHER LESIONS

Adding interest to this group of benign small bowel tumors is their infrequent association with abnormalities of skin, mucous membranes, sub-

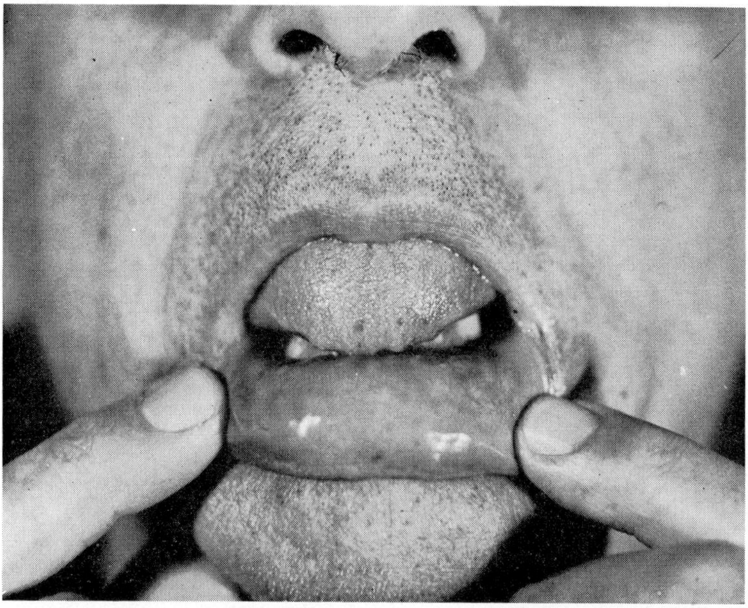

Figure 4–7. Case of Osler-Weber-Rendu syndrome. Note telangiectasia of mucous membranes of lips.

cutaneous tissues, and bone. Frequently these associations are highlighted by an inherited mendelian dominant trait. Peutz[46] and Jeghers[23] have described a syndrome of pigmented spots on the oral mucosa, the external lips, or the fingers associated with multiple adenomatous polyps of the small bowel. Multiple neurofibromatosis of the small bowel has been seen in patients with von Recklinghausen's disease. Hashemian[19] has described multiple fibromas of the small bowel occurring in association with scattered areas of pigmentation on the body in a mother, son, and daughter. The hereditary hemorrhagic telangiectasia syndrome (Osler-Weber-Rendu) involving the small bowel and mucous membranes of the eye, nose, and mouth is likewise an unusual and fascinating condition (Fig. 4–7).[37, 41, 52] The association of soft tissue tumors and intestinal polyposis (occasionally in small intestine), called Gardner's syndrome, has also been noted.[15]

ADENOMATOUS POLYPS

We refer to adenomatous polyps as intraluminal projections of the mucous membrane and submucosa, the projection consisting of a central fibrovascular core surrounded by acini with varying degrees of differentiation. Glandular cells must be present in the epithelial layer for them to be distinguished as adenomatous polyps. River et al.[53] found this the most common benign tumor. However, Gannon et al.[14] separated out a large group

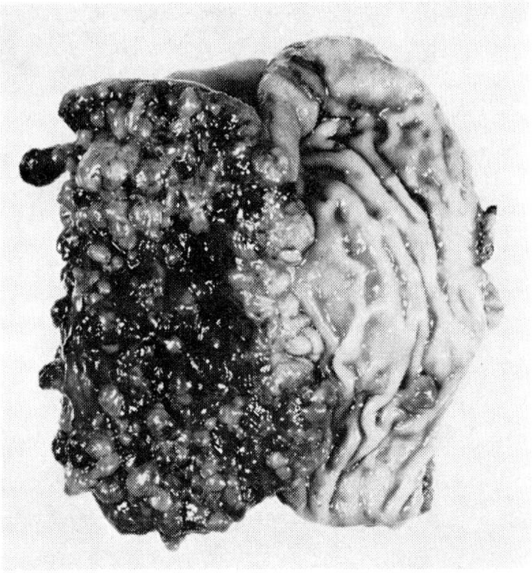

Figure 4–8. Villous adenomatous polyp of ileum. This patient had multiple polyps (benign) of large and small intestine.

of hamartomatous polyps and gastric heterotopic polyps, leaving only a few true adenomatous polyps in the Mayo Clinic experience. As with the other benign tumors, the most common symptoms were related to obstruction, with bleeding being second in frequency. Adenomatous polyps of the small intestine may be single; they may be multiple, involving a short segment of the small bowel or the entire small bowel; or they may be associated with adenomatosis of the entire abdominal gastrointestinal tract (Fig. 4–8).[50]

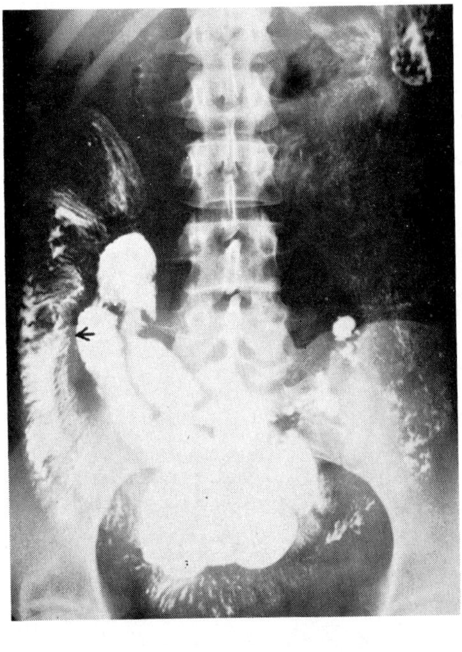

Figure 4–9. Barium study showing villous polyp of jejunum which on excision had a focus of adenocarcinoma. (From Heffernon, E. W.: Gastroenterology *42*:61, January, 1962.)

Occasionally, the condition is familial, as when it is associated with adenomatosis of the colon or is part of the Peutz-Jeghers syndrome.[6] The possibility of malignant degeneration is known, but the exact incidence is not available (Fig. 4–9).[20, 23, 25]

Because of their frequent tendency to bleed or to serve as the leading point of an intussusception, and because of their known ability to undergo malignant degeneration, the elective removal of single or multiple asymptomatic small intestinal polyps is justifiable and advisable. The exceptions to this generality are patients whose general condition and life expectancy are unsuitable for elective procedures. In addition, if multiple polyps so extensively involve the small bowel that their removal by resection would not leave enough small intestine for normal function, elective surgical treatment is not desirable.

When the complications of obstruction and hemorrhage are present, either the polyps must be excised or the involved bowel must be resected. Since polyps are the most common cause of intussusception in the adult, and since it may be impossible to palpate them after reduction of an intussusception, resection of the involved bowel, or at least an enterotomy, is mandatory.

PEUTZ-JEGHERS SYNDROME

The Peutz-Jeghers syndrome was first noted by Peutz in 1921[46] and recalled by Jeghers in 1949.[23] It is characterized by multiple adenomatous polyps of the gastrointestinal tract, most often involving the small intestine, associated with melanin spots on the oral mucosa, lips, and digits. Fifty-nine cases were collected by River et al.[53] through December 1954, and the number in the literature had risen to over a hundred by 1963.[12] The condition is familial and appears to be inherited as a mendelian dominant trait; however, sporadic cases may occasionally occur.

The course of these patients is marked by repeated episodes of obstruction from intussusception and periods of melena of minor to major severity. Doubt as to the premalignant nature of the small intestinal polyps of the Peutz-Jeghers syndrome has been raised by Bartholomew et al.[3] In their opinion these polyps are hamartomatous and are not premalignant. They further pointed out that there had not been one proved case of metastasis from a Peutz-Jeghers polyp of the small bowel. Of interest is a recent report of Warren et al.[67] of a patient with this syndrome in whom a malignant duodenal polyp with metastases was found. In the treatment of the intestinal complications of this syndrome, extreme caution must be exercised to avoid massive resection of the bowel. There is a real danger of leaving the patient a cripple from the short bowel syndrome.

Table 4–6. Benign and Malignant Vascular Lesions of the Small Bowel*

Benign
Telangiectasis (hereditary and nonhereditary)
Hemangioma
Capillary
Mixed
Cavernous
Malignant
Hemangioendothelioma
Benign metastasizing hemangioma
Kaposi's sarcoma
Angiosarcoma

*Adapted from Gentry, R. W., et. al.: Internat. Abstr. Surg. *88:*282 (1949); *in* Surg. Gynec. & Obst. (Apr.) 1949.

VASCULAR TUMORS

An extensive review of vascular malformations and tumors of the gastrointestinal tract has been made by Gentry et al.,[16] who reported 136 vascular tumors of the small intestine, 87 percent of which were benign. Nys and Buyssens[40] recently reviewed cavernous hemangiomas. As mentioned previously, hemorrhage is a prominent symptom of this group of cases, although obstruction is common. At operation, the differential diagnosis includes chylangiomas and chronic congestion of the portal system. Transillumination of the bowel is suggested as an aid in visualizing small tumors, and resection of the involved segment is the treatment of choice. Occasionally because of the extent of the disease, this is impossible. The Osler[41]-Weber-Rendu[52] syndrome (Fig. 4–7) with multiple telangiectasia is an example.[37] Under these circumstances, replacement transfusion is about the only possible treatment. Snake venom, rutin, and radiation have been tried with indifferent success. The pathologic classification used by Gentry et al.[16] is shown in Table 4–6. A more detailed consideration of the subject is found in Chapter Fourteen.

OTHER TYPES OF BENIGN TUMORS

The mesenchymal tissue tumors, lipomas, fibromas, and myomas follow the epithelial tumors in frequency.[53] Their clinical characteristics, diagnosis, and treatment do not differ appreciably from other tumors. Starr and Dockerty,[62] in 1955, reviewed the smooth muscle tumors extensively.

A wide variety of tumors has been reported in Meckel's diverticula.[21, 38, 60] This unusual location for tumors is of importance as a leading point for intussusception, a source of occult bleeding, or for their malignant characteristics.

REPORT OF CASES

Case 1. Fibroma of the Small Bowel. A 30-year-old woman was first seen at the clinic in November 1942. She had noted for four months previously a small mass, the size of an egg, in her left mid-abdomen. Her complaints at that time were related to flatulence and a feeling of fullness in the abdomen.

Physical examination revealed a firm, round, smooth, movable mass the size of a volley ball in the patient's abdomen. Routine laboratory studies were within normal limits. The plain film of the abdomen and the barium enema roentgenogram showed only a large soft tissue mass.

The patient was taken to surgery and at laparotomy a large solid tumor was found in the mesentery adjacent to and involving the wall of the mid-jejunum. The jejunum which traversed the tumor was not obstructed. The tumor was resected with approximately 24 inches of jejunum, and a side-to-side anastomosis was performed.

Microscopic examination of the tumor, which weighed 1840 gm., revealed it to be a fibroma. Convalescence from this procedure was uneventful.

This case illustrates the huge size that benign tumors of the small intestine may attain. At laparotomy the surgeon's diagnosis was adenocarcinoma. Several nodes were palpable in the mesentery of the involved intestine. In spite of this clinical impression, this benign lesion was resected. Every attempt must be made by the surgeon to remove visible disease, regardless of his gross tissue diagnosis.

Case 2. A 60-year-old woman came to the clinic for evaluation of her chronic bronchiectasis. On routine examination a mass was felt in the right flank. On questioning, she admitted chronic diarrhea and stated that her friends had noted intermittent, transient, facial flushing. A tentative diagnosis was made of carcinoid syndrome.

Roentgenologic examination of the gastrointestinal tract revealed a soft tissue mass, approximately 12 cm. in diameter, in the right mid-abdomen overlying the iliac crest.

Further questioning of the patient revealed that these episodes of sensation of warmth never lasted more than five minutes; she described the flushing as a "surging" into her face and neck. They actually were first noticed by her nephew who remarked on the extreme redness of her face; at the time she was having lunch and experiencing a warm sensation. Since the initial episode, the flushing had been variable in occurrence but might average two episodes a day. They were related only to eating and the recumbent position.

The quantitative 5-hydroxy-indoleacetic acid in the 24-hour urine specimen ranged from 24 to 111 mg. per 24 hours. Initially, approximately one third of the quantitative serotonin determinations were negative.

The patient was taken to surgery, and at laparotomy a polypoid lesion approximately 2.0 cm. in diameter was found in the terminal portion of the ileum. There were multiple, large metastatic nodes in the mesentery of the distal ileum as well as multiple metastatic nodules of a yellowish tinge spread diffusely in both lobes of the liver.

This case is presented to give the detailed characteristics of flushing and the other clinical stigmata of the carcinoid syndrome.

Case 3. A 30-year-old woman was first seen at the clinic complaining of vomiting of 15 months' duration. This vomiting was intermittent in that it occurred seemingly at three-week intervals. However, for the month previous to her first visit to the clinic, it had been a daily occurrence. She also noted generalized abdominal cramps with visible "bunching" in her abdomen and had reportedly lost 42 pounds. Her appetite and strength had been poor.

On physical examination there was slight tenderness in the right upper quadrant. The routine laboratory tests were within normal limits, and the roentgenogram of the abdomen was normal. However, the upper gastrointestinal series revealed that the distal small bowel was dilated.

On July 22, 1941, the patient was taken to surgery, and at laparotomy an obstructing lesion was found approximately 30 cm. proximal to the ileocecal valve. This lesion was annular and 3.7 cm. in length. A wedge of the small intestine was resected with removal of adjacent mesentery, and an end-to-end anastomosis was performed. The pathologist reported the tumor to be an adenocarcinoma.

Postoperative recovery was uneventful and the patient was well at the time of her last visit in May 1956.

This case illustrates the common complaints of pain, vomiting, and weight loss associated with a chronic, partially obstructing tumor of the small intestine.

Case 4. This patient was first seen at the clinic in 1935, at which time he was only 19 years of age. He complained of crampy, lower abdominal pain, melena, and weight loss. Two laparotomies had been performed elsewhere that year, at which time an appendectomy and removal of a polyp of the transverse colon with side-to-side ileocolostomy had been performed. Barium studies and proctoscopic examination revealed polyposis of the colon. Resection of the large intestine with ileosigmoidostomy was performed.

In the period from 1935 to 1955 he was seen on several occasions in this clinic for fulguration of rectal polyps. From time to time during this period he had noted diarrheal type stools, up to five per day, with a fluctuating body weight.

In August 1955, the patient was admitted to the hospital with a two-week history of severe upper gastrointestinal bleeding. An upper gastrointestinal x-ray series was consistent with an infiltrating neoplasm involving most of the stomach, and multiple polyps were noted in the distal small bowel. The patient was submitted to laparotomy in 1955, and a subtotal gastrectomy was performed for multiple polyposis of the stomach. Evidence of malignant disease was not found. Polyps were present in all portions of the stomach and several were left behind in the gastric stump.

In 1958, on an upper gastrointestinal x-ray series, diffuse polyposis of the distal ileum was noted. He continued to visit the clinic as an outpatient at regular intervals at which time fulguration of recurrent polyps of the rectal segment was accomplished.

In May 1961, the ileorectal anastomosis was resected with reanastomosis. On examination of the open small bowel, multiple small polyps were seen throughout the entire length of the small intestine.

Throughout all these years his main complaints have been melena with occasional hematemesis of bright red blood. To date, there is no evidence that any of the polyps have undergone malignant degeneration.

This patient had diffuse gastrointestinal adenomatosis. Fortunately, malignant degeneration has not been noted in any of his polyps. His long-term condition has been marked throughout these years with bleeding and anemia.

Case 5. This patient was first seen at the clinic in July 1935 at the age of 22. At that time he had noted hematemesis that had responded to iron-liver therapy as administered by his local physician. An upper gastrointestinal series revealed only a possible duodenal ulcer and an apparently enlarged spleen.

On August 7, 1935, he was taken to surgery, at which time the small intestine appeared hyperemic. The veins throughout the mesentery and the superficial and deep veins of the small bowel wall were greatly dilated with blotchy erythemic areas scattered throughout the bowel. The small intestinal wall was thickened and doughy. The colon had dilated veins on its surface and in the mesentery, but was of normal color and thickness. The spleen was enlarged to four times normal size. No definitive procedure was done at that time.

Since this patient's first visit in 1935, he has been seen in this clinic on numerous occasions and has been hospitalized for a total of 16 admissions. In the 28 years following his initial visit, he has received well over 100 units of whole blood. Multiple surgical procedures have been performed for hemorrhage, resulting in the excision of a total of some 240 cm. of small bowel. The pathologic diagnosis was ectasia or hemangioma of the submucosal blood vessels. These lesions ranged from 1 to 3 mm. in diameter. There was no pulsation in these structures.

This case illustrates the very rare condition of small intestinal hemangiomatosis. The patient has been kept alive by the use of transfusions and selected resective procedures when hemorrhage became alarming.

SUMMARY

Tumors of the small intestine present a wide spectrum of pathologic types. Approximately 35 varieties are reported in the world literature. The most common types are adenocarcinomas, lymphomas, carcinoids, and the benign lesions.

In autopsy series, benign lesions outnumber malignant tumors. In clinical series the malignant varieties are most numerous. Usually, these tumors are found in older patients, and there is no sex preponderance.

The symptoms and findings on physical examination in patients with small bowel tumors are related to their tendency to obstruct or bleed. The precise clinical diagnosis can often be made on radiologic examination of the small intestine. However, this examination is not always successful in demonstrating these tumors. The success rate appears to be proportional to the care with which the examination is conducted.

The adenocarcinomas, lymphomas, carcinoid tumors, carcinoid syndrome, adenomatous polyps, and vascular tumors are discussed in some detail.

REFERENCES

1. Alrich, E. M., Blank, R. H., and Fomon, J. J.: Primary tumors of the small intestine. Am. J. Surg. *99:*33–39 (Jan.) 1960.
2. Aschoff, L., Editor: Pathologische Anatomie; ein Lehrbuch für Studierende und Ärzte. 3. Aufl., 2 v. Jena, Gustav Fischer, 1911.
3. Bartholomew, L. G., Dahlin, D. C., and Waugh, J. M.: Intestinal polyposis associated with mucocutaneous melanin pigmentation (Peutz-Jeghers syndrome); review of literature and report of six cases with special reference to pathologic findings. Gastroenterology *32:*434–451 (Mar.) 1957.
4. Bernstein, J. S., and Chey, W. Y.: Small bowel tumors; a clinical study of 109 cases. J. Mt. Sinai Hosp. *25:*1–28 (Jan.-Feb.) 1958.
5. Botsford, T. W., Crowe, P., and Crocker, D. W.: Tumors of the small intestine. A review of experience with 115 cases including a report of a rare case of malignant hemangioendothelioma. Am. J. Surg. *103:*358–365 (Mar.) 1962.
6. Calabro, J. J.: Hereditable multiple polyposis syndromes of the gastrointestinal tract. Am. J. Med. *33:*276–281 (Aug.) 1962.
7. Cameron, A. L.: Primary malignancy of the jejunum and ileum. Ann. Surg. *108:*203–220 (Aug.) 1938.

8. Cattell, R. B., Warren, K. W., and Au, F. T. C.: Periampullary carcinomas; diagnosis and surgical management. S. Clin. North America *39:*781–798 (June) 1959.
9. Crile, G.: Discussion of Wilson, H., and Butterick, O. D., Jr.: Massive liver resection for control of severe vasomotor reactions secondary to malignant carcinoid. Ann. Surg. *149:*651 (May) 1959.
10. Davis, R. B.: Observations on the occurrence and significance of serotonin in carcinoid tumors. Am. J. Path. *41:*693–709 (Dec.) 1962.
11. Davis, R. B., Alexander, C. S., and Adicoff, A.: Metabolic studies in carcinoid syndrome: observations on use of a-methyl DOPA, isonicotinic acid hydrazide and selective tryptophan deficiency. Metabolism *10:*1035–1044 (Dec.) 1961.
12. Farmer, R. G., Hawk, W. A., and Turnbull, R. B., Jr.: The spectrum of the Peutz-Jeghers syndrome: Report of three cases. Am. J. Digest. Dis. *8:*953–961 (Nov.) 1963.
13. Gall, E. A., and Mallory, T. B.: Malignant lymphoma: a clinicopathologic survey of 618 cases. Am. J. Path. *18:*381–430 (May) 1942.
14. Gannon, P. G., Dahlin, D. C., Bartholomew, L. G., and Beahrs, O. H.: Polypoid glandular tumors of the small intestine. Surg. Gynec. & Obst. *114:*666–672 (June) 1962.
15. Gardner, E. J., and Richards, R. C.: Multiple cutaneous and subcutaneous lesions occurring simultaneously with hereditary polyposis and osteomatosis. Am. J. Human Genet. *5:*139–147 (June) 1953.
16. Gentry, R. W., Dockerty, M. B., and Clagett, O. T.: Collective review; vascular malformations and vascular tumors of gastrointestinal tract. Internat. Abstr. Surg. *88:*281–323, 1949; *in* Surg. Gynec. & Obst. (Apr.) 1949.
17. Goble, A. J., Hay, D. R., and Sandler, M.: 5-Hydroxytryptamine metabolism in acquired heart-disease associated with argentaffin carcinoma; preliminary communication. Lancet *2:*1016–1017 (Nov. 12) 1955.
18. Golden, R., and Morales, P. L.: Radiological examination in organic diseases of small intestine. J.A.M.A. *153:*1431–1433 (Dec. 19) 1953.
19. Hashemian, H.: Familial fibromatosis. Brit. J. Surg. *40:*346–350 (Jan.) 1953.
20. Heffernon, E. W., Metcalfe, O., and Schwarz, H. J., Jr.: Polyposis of the small and large bowel with carcinoma in a villous polyp of the jejunum. Gastroenterology *42:*60–62 (Jan.) 1962.
21. Hill, F. A., and Janelli, D. E.: Malignant tumors originating in Meckel's diverticulum; case report of leiomyosarcoma and review of literature. Am. J. Surg. *85:*525–528 (Apr.) 1953.
22. Isler, P., and Hedinger, C.: Metastasierendes Dunndarmcarcinoid mit schweren, vorwiegend das rechte Herz betreffenden Klappenfehlern und Pulmonal-stenose—ein eigenartiger Symptomenkomplex? Schweiz. med. Wchnschr. *83:*4–7 (Jan. 3) 1953.
23. Jeghers, H., McKusick, V. A., and Katz, K. H.: Generalized intestinal polyposis and melanin spots of oral mucosa, lips and digits; syndrome of diagnostic significance. New England J. Med. *241:*993–1005 (Dec. 22) 1949; 1031–1036 (Dec. 29) 1949.
24. Jenkinson, E. L., Pfisterer, W. H., and Seitz, E. R.: Primary tumors of small intestine. Radiology *55:*12–19 (July) 1950.
25. Joergenson, E. J., and Weibel, L. A.: Study of small bowel tumors with special emphasis on clinical aspects. California Med. *75:*395–399 (Dec.) 1951.
26. Keats, T. E., and Sakai, H. Q.: Evaluation of sources of error in the roentgenologic diagnosis of neoplasms of the small intestine. Gastroenterology *29:*554–562 (Oct.) 1955.
27. Likely, D. S., Lisa, J. R., Stitch, M. H., and Stein, H. D.: Primary malignant disease of small bowel. Arch. Int. Med. *82:*206–216 (Aug.) 1948.
28. Lubarsch, O.: Ueber den primären Krebs des Ileum, nebst Bemerkungen über das gleichzeitige Vorkommen von Krebs und Tuberculose. Arch. path. Anat. *111:*280–317, 1888.
29. MacDonald, R. A.: A study of 356 carcinoids of the gastrointestinal tract; report of four new cases of the carcinoid syndrome. Am. J. Med. *21:*867–878 (Dec.) 1956.
30. Masson, P.: Carcinoids (argentaffin-cell tumors) and nerve hyperplasia of appendicular mucosa. Am. J. Path. *4:*181–212 (May) 1928.
31. Mayo, C. W.: Malignancy of the small intestine. West. J. Surg. *48:*403–407 (July) 1940.
32. Mayo, C. W., and Nettrour, W. S.: Carcinoma of the jejunum. Surg. Gynec. & Obst. *65:*303–309 (Sept.) 1937.
33. McKusick, V. A.: Carcinoid cardiovascular disease. Bull. Johns Hopkins Hosp. *98:*13–36 (Jan.) 1956.
34. Meissner, W.: Quoted in Warren, K. W., and Littlefield, J. B. (Ref. 66, p. 737).

35. Mengel, C. E., Weaver, W., Holloway, L., and Anlyan, W. G.: Adjuvant therapy of malignant carcinoid syndrome. Surgery *54:*182–190 (July) 1963.
36. Moertel, C. G., Sauer, W. G., Dockerty, M. B., and Baggenstoss, A. H.: Life history of the carcinoid tumor of the small intestine. Cancer *14:*901–912 (Sept.-Oct.) 1961.
37. Monroe, L. S., and Spencer, F. M.: The clinical significance of hereditary hemorrhagic telangiectasia. Gastroenterology *38:*906–911 (June) 1960.
38. Moore, R. M., and Parsons, W. H.: Carcinoma of Meckel's diverticulum; report of case with summary review of literature. Arch. Surg. *67:*939–942 (Dec.) 1953.
39. Mosenthal, W. T.: Resection of massive liver metastases in the malignant carcinoid syndrome. Review and report of a case. S. Clin. North America *43:*1253–1262 (Oct.) 1963.
40. Nys, A., and Buyssens, N.: Diffuse cavernous hemangiomatosis of the small intestine. Gastroenterology *45:*663–666 (Nov.) 1963.
41. Osler, W.: On a family form of recurring epistaxis, associated with multiple telangiectases of the skin and mucous membranes. Bull. Johns Hopkins Hosp. *12:*333–337 (Nov.) 1901.
42. Page, I. H.: Serotonin (5-hydroxytryptamine); the last four years. Physiol. Rev. *38:*277–335 (Apr.) 1958.
43. Page, I. H., and McCubbin, J. W.: Variable arterial pressure response to serotonin in laboratory animals and man. Circulation Res. *1:*354–362 (July) 1953.
44. Page, I. H., Corcoran, A. C., Udenfriend, S., Sjoerdsma, A., and Weissbach, H.: Argentaffinoma as endocrine tumour. Lancet *1:*198–199 (Jan. 22) 1955.
45. Pernow, B., and Waldenström, J.: Determination of 5-hydroxytryptamine, 5-hydroxyindole acetic acid and histamine in thirty-three cases of carcinoid tumor (argentaffinoma). Am. J. Med. *23:*16–25 (July) 1957.
46. Peutz, J. L. A.: On a very remarkable case of familial polyposis of the mucous membrane of the intestinal tract and nasopharynx accompanied by peculiar pigmentations of the skin and mucous membrane. Nederl. Maandschr. v. Geneesk. *10:*134–146, 1921.
47. Postlethwait, R. W.: Gastrointestinal carcinoid tumors. A review. Postgrad. Med. *40:*445–454 (Oct.) 1966.
48. Rankin, F. W., and Newell, C. E.: Benign tumors of the small intestine. Report of twenty-four cases. Surg. Gynec. & Obst. *57:*501–506 (Oct.) 1933.
49. Ransom, W. B.: A case of primary carcinoma of the ileum. Lancet *2:*1020–1023 (Nov. 15) 1890.
50. Ravitch, M. M.: Polypoid adenomatosis of entire gastro-intestinal tract. Ann. Surg. *128:*283–298 (Aug.) 1948.
51. Reed, M. L., Kuipers, F. M., Vaitkevicius, V. K., Clark, M. D., Drake, E. H., and Eyler, W. R.: Treatment of disseminated carcinoid tumors including hepatic-artery catheterization. New England J. Med. *269:*1005–1010 (Nov. 7) 1963.
52. Rendu, M.: Épistaxis répétées chez un sujet porteur de petits angiomes cutanés et muqueux. Bull. et mém. Soc. méd. d. hôp. de Paris. *13:*731–733 (Oct. 23) 1896.
53. River, L., Silverstein, J., and Tope, J. W.: Collective review: benign neoplasms of small intestine; critical comprehensive review with reports of 20 new cases. Internat. Abstr. Surg. *102:*1–38, 1956; *in* Surg. Gynec. & Obst. (Jan.) 1956.
54. Rochlin, D. B., and Longmire, W. P., Jr.: Primary tumors of the small intestine. Surgery *50:*586–592 (Oct.) 1961.
55. Schatzki, R.: Small intestinal enema. Am. J. Roentgenol. *50:*743–751 (Dec.) 1943.
56. Shallow, T. A., Eger, S. A., and Carty, J. B.: Primary malignant disease of the small intestine. Am. J. Surg. *69:*372–383 (Sept.) 1945.
57. Sjoerdsma, A., Weissbach, H., and Udenfriend, S.: Simple test for diagnosis of metastatic carcinoid (argentaffinoma). J.A.M.A. *159:*397 (Sept. 24) 1955.
58. Sjoerdsma, A., Weissbach, H., Terry, L. L., and Udenfriend, S.: Further observations on patients with malignant carcinoid. Am. J. Med. *23:*5–15 (July) 1957.
59. Snow, P. J. D., Lennard-Jones, J. E., Curzon, G., and Stacey, R. S.: Humoral effects of metastasising carcinoid tumours. Lancet *2:*1004–1009 (Nov. 12) 1955.
60. Southam, J. A.: Primary malignant tumours of the jejunum and ileum. Brit. J. Surg. *50:*393–399 (Jan.) 1963.
61. Stanford, W. R., Davis, J. E., Gunter, J. U., and Hobart, S. G., Jr.: Bronchial adenoma (carcinoid type) with solitary metastasis and associated functioning carcinoid syndrome. South. M. J. *51:*449–454 (Apr.) 1958.

62. Starr, G. F., and Dockerty, M. B.: Leiomyomas and leiomyosarcomas of small intestine. Cancer *8:*101–111 (Jan.-Feb.) 1955.
63. Stone, H. H., and Donnelly, C. C.: The anesthetic significance of serotonin secreting carcinoid tumors. Anesthesiology *21:*203–212 (Mar.-Apr.) 1960.
64. Strohl, E. L., and Diffenbaugh, W. G.: Primary tumors of the small bowel. Arch. Surg. *74:*709–718 (May) 1957.
65. Thorson, A., Biörck, G., Björkman, G., and Waldenström, J.: Malignant carcinoid of small intestine with metastases to liver, valvular disease of right side of heart (pulmonary stenosis and tricuspid regurgitation without septal defects), peripheral vasomotor symptoms, bronchoconstriction, and unusual type of cyanosis; clinical and pathologic syndrome. Am. Heart J. *47:*795–817 (June) 1954.
66. Warren, K. W., and Littlefield, J. B.: Malignant lymphomas of the gastrointestinal tract. S. Clin. North America *35:*735–746 (June) 1955.
67. Warren, K. W., Kune, G. A., and Poulantzas, J. K.: Peutz-Jeghers syndrome with carcinoma of the duodenum and jejunum. Lahey Clin. Found. Bull. *14:*97–102, 1965.
68. Weber, H. M., and Kirklin, B. R.: Roentgenologic manifestations of tumors of the small intestine. Am. J. Roentgenol. *47:*243–253 (Feb.) 1942.
69. Weibel, L. A., Joergenson, E. J., and Keasbey, L. E.: Clinical study of small bowel tumors; report of 165 lesions. Am. J. Gastroenterol. *21:*466–477 (June) 1954.
70. Williams, M. J., Sutherland, D. H., and Clark, C. G.: Lymphosarcoma of the small intestine with malabsorption syndrome and pneumatosis intestinalis: Report of a case with peroral jejunal biopsy. Gastroenterology *45:*550–557 (Oct.) 1963.
71. Wilson, H., Storer, E. H., and Star, F. J.: Carcinoid tumors. A study of seventy-eight cases. Am. J. Surg. *105:*35–39 (Jan.) 1963.

Chapter Five

INFLAMMATORY DISEASE

REGIONAL ENTERITIS

Regional enteritis (Crohn's disease) is the most common inflammatory disease of the small intestine. It is of unknown etiology and there is no specific medical treatment for it.

A case with findings similar to regional enteritis is said to have been reported by Morgagni in 1769,[53] and a paper on thickening and stricture of the terminal ileum was read before the College of Physicians of London in 1806.[17] Dalziel,[22] in 1913, added a case to the six then reported in the literature. In 1923, Wilensky and Moschcowitz[57] distinguished between enteritis and tuberculosis, and reviewed four cases of granulomatous ileitis, one of which was regional enteritis.

Regional enteritis was first accepted as a clinical entity when Crohn[19] reported 13 cases in 1932. Bargen,[3] in discussing Crohn's paper, pointed out that the disease was not always confined to the terminal ileum. Crohn then changed the name from regional ileitis to regional enteritis. It is of interest that British surgeons still prefer to call it Crohn's disease rather than regional enteritis.

Undoubtedly, many times the diagnosis is not made because in some patients the disease develops and subsides spontaneously. In other patients, it may have an acute onset, develop rapidly, and simulate acute appendicitis with perforation. In the typical patient, the disease is slowly progressive until obstruction of the small bowel, perforation, or the development of internal or external fistulas makes surgery imperative.

The treatment of regional enteritis is one of the unsolved problems in abdominal surgery. In at least one of every four patients treated surgically the disease recurs. In many instances, the abdominal disease is so extensive that it taxes the skill of any surgeon.

INCIDENCE

Judging from the medical literature, regional enteritis was relatively rare when it was first described in 1932. The experience at large clinics would indicate that the frequency of the disease is increasing.[2, 13, 53] We do not know how much of the apparent increase in incidence is the result of better recognition of this condition. Because regional enteritis is seldom fatal, it is not surprising that it did not become well known long ago in the autopsy room. Until recently, it was almost unknown in Latin America and the Orient. It appears to be more common in Jewish people and less common in Negroes. A familial susceptibility is unusual, but it does occur. Bockus[9] has reported 22 families in which regional enteritis attacked more than one person in the same family for a total of 49 cases. He believes that the familial incidence exceeds that of ulcerative colitis and that genetic factors rather than infectious agents are responsible.

PATHOGENESIS

Many pathologists, including our own, believe that regional enteritis begins as a granulomatous lymphangitis in the mesentery of the small intestine[54, 55, 56] (Fig. 5–1). This produces obstruction of the lymphatic vessels in the mesentery, which in turn results in edema and thickening of the intestinal wall. As the disease persists, this leads to fibrosis, narrowing, and eventual obstruction of the bowel lumen. Ulceration of the mucosa first de-

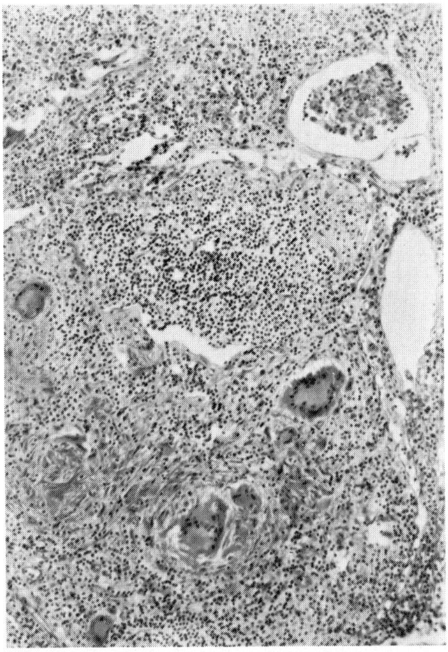

Figure 5–1. Lymph node from mesentery of small bowel involved with regional enteritis showing granulomatous lymphangitis. (From Colcock, B. P.: Regional Enteritis. Current Problems in Surgery. Chicago, Year Book Medical Publishers, Inc., 1965, p. 5.)

velops in the mesenteric border and then extends in an irregular manner, leaving isolated islands of intact mucosa. Once ulceration develops, the factor of secondary infection is added. Perforation may occur, leading to an abscess or a fistula between loops of small bowel, or between the small bowel and the colon, the vagina, and occasionally the bladder. If an operation has been performed, a fistula may develop between the bowel and the skin at the site of the incision.

Recently, the origin of the disease in the mesentery of the small bowel has been questioned by other pathologists who believe that the disease actually begins in the submucosa of the intestinal wall.[39] This causes edema and telangiectasis of the bowel wall, and later produces striking changes in the mesentery. The fibrosis, granulomatous formations, and so forth are thought to be secondary to the initial pathologic changes in the submucosa.

Grossly, the bowel is edematous and hyperemic, with the consistency of a rubber garden hose. The serosa is often obscured by the extension of the mesenteric fat that may cover all but the antimesenteric border. The mesentery is greatly thickened with enlarged lymph nodes that may form huge masses, often several centimeters in diameter. As the lumen of the bowel is decreased because of the inflammatory reaction, the proximal portion of the bowel becomes hypertrophied. Exudate may be present on the surface of the involved bowel, and much turbid fluid may be found in the peritoneal cavity, depending upon the acuteness of the inflammatory reaction.

On opening the bowel, the surgeon may find the mucosal layer completely destroyed at the point of maximum involvement. The typical ulceration will be found just proximal to this area. The marked thickening of the bowel wall is the most striking finding (Fig. 5–2). The muscular layer seems

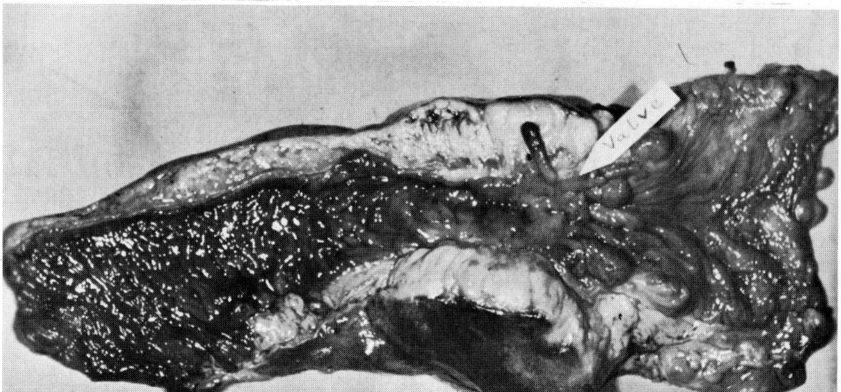

Figure 5–2. Resected terminal ileum and cecum showing marked thickening of the ileum with loss of the villous mucosal pattern due to regional enteritis which stops abruptly at the ileocecal valve. (From Colcock, B. P.: Regional Enteritis. Current Problems in Surgery. Chicago, Year Book Medical Publishers, Inc., 1965, p. 7.)

to be relatively resistant to the disease until it is penetrated by the secondary suppurative process. On microscopic examination, the outstanding feature is the extensive fibroblastic proliferation that has occurred (Fig. 5–3). Since this far exceeds that necessary for repair of damaged tissue, it suggests an altered tissue reaction to the causative agent. What this agent is, no one knows. The fact that the disease so often stops abruptly at the junction of the ileum with the colon suggests that the colon possesses an inherent resistance that the small bowel does not have. That the terminal small bowel is usually involved might be because the specific agent increases in quantity or toxicity as it progresses down the bowel. The latest theory is that regional enteritis may be an autoimmune disease, but as yet there is no proof of this. It may be that there is no one specific cause.

Clinically, the disease involves the terminal ileum in 9 of 10 patients. This is the reason that Crohn at first called it regional ileitis, a term still used by many physicians. Fifteen percent of these patients have so-called skip areas in other parts of the gastrointestinal tract.[14] The second most common site is the proximal ileum, and the third is the jejunum. The disease may affect the duodenum, the stomach, and even the esophagus, and frequently involves the cecal wall and a part of the ascending colon. Rarely, it appears in segments of the remaining colon and rectum.

One of the most intriguing aspects of regional enteritis is its strong tendency to develop just proximal to the junction of the small bowel and colon. Recurrent disease after resection or bypass behaves in an even more

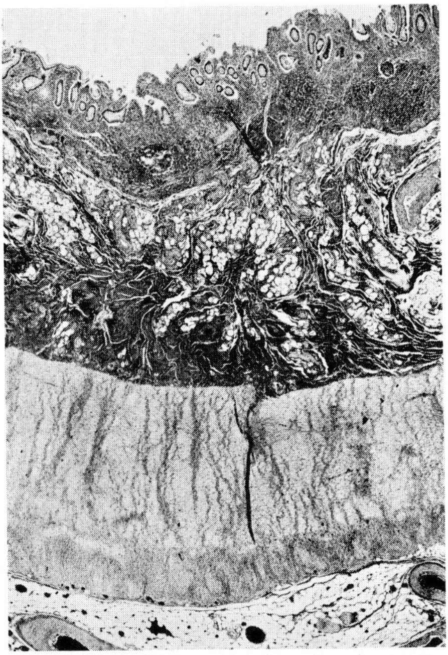

Figure 5–3. Microscopic features of regional enteritis showing extensive fibroblastic proliferation in submucosal layers. (From Colcock, B. P.: Regional Enteritis. Current Problems in Surgery. Chicago, Year Book Medical Publishers, Inc., 1965, p. 8.)

striking manner: almost invariably it recurs just proximal to the ileocolic anastomosis.

ASSOCIATED DISEASE

Regional enteritis is frequently associated with other gastrointestinal diseases, the most common in our experience are cholelithiasis (10 percent), duodenal ulcer (8 percent), and ulcerative colitis (8 percent).[13]

Ulcerative colitis also is a disease of unknown etiology. Most pathologists believe that ulcerative colitis and regional enteritis are not the same disease. If this is true, they can coexist, and when a patient has both regional enteritis and ulcerative colitis, he presents an extremely serious problem from the point of view of treatment. Like patients with regional enteritis, ulcerative colitis patients frequently require surgery either because a complication of the disease has developed or because the disease has become refractory to medical treatment. The only satisfactory surgical treatment for most of these patients is an ileostomy and colectomy. If, in addition, enteritis of the ileum develops that requires resection, the patient may be left with a short segment of small bowel and no colon or rectum. He then leads a precarious existence. Any abnormal fluid or electrolyte loss, unless corrected promptly, may be fatal.

In 1961, we reported 39 patients with both ulcerative colitis and regional enteritis; the mortality rate in this small group was 25 percent.[15] Both diseases occurred primarily in the young adult, but regional enteritis had a somewhat earlier onset. In 32 of the 39 patients, symptoms of regional enteritis developed first; in five patients, both conditions developed at approximately the same time; and in two patients, the ulcerative colitis developed first. With careful management, however, patients having both enteritis and ulcerative colitis can be salvaged. Almost all of the 75 percent of patients who survived were restored to a normal, active life.

Unlike patients with ulcerative colitis, regional enteritis is seldom, if ever, associated with the later development of carcinoma. Although cancer of the colon occurs in 5 to 10 percent of our patients with ulcerative colitis of long standing (10 years or more), we have not seen carcinoma of the small bowel in a patient with regional enteritis.

CLINICAL FINDINGS

Regional enteritis is primarily a disease of the young adult.[14] We have had patients as young as 10 years and as old as 79 years who have required surgical treatment for regional enteritis. Sixty-two percent of our patients were less than 30 years of age when their symptoms began. It should not be forgotten, however, that regional enteritis does develop in patients who are middle-aged or older. Five to 8 percent of our patients were more than

50 years of age when the disease began. Therefore, it must be considered, even in the older patient, in the differential diagnosis of an inflammatory lesion of the abdomen.

Regional enteritis is somewhat more common in males.[14] Conversely, we find that recurrent disease is more likely to develop in the female than in the male.

The characteristic symptoms of regional enteritis are abdominal pain and diarrhea. These symptoms are usually associated with a low-grade fever, leukocytosis, and tenderness in the right lower quadrant. As a rule, the abdominal pain is periumbilical in location, cramplike, and aggravated by taking food. Unlike ulcerative colitis, regional enteritis does not commonly cause gross rectal bleeding unless the colon is involved. However, anemia is likely to develop in these patients because of occult bleeding and malnutrition.

DIAGNOSIS

When the onset of regional enteritis is acute, it must be distinguished from acute appendicitis. The pain in the right lower quadrant, the localized tenderness, fever, and leukocytosis present a diagnostic problem. In both regional enteritis and acute appendicitis, a tender palpable mass may be present in the right lower portion of the abdomen. In this situation the history is often helpful. If there has been a loss of weight and if fever and abdominal pain have been present for a considerable period of time, enteritis should be suspected. The same is true if there is a history of frequent, fatty, foul-smelling, diarrheal stools and occult blood. A persistent enterocutaneous fistula in the right lower quadrant usually indicates regional enteritis, although it could be the result of pathologic changes in the appendix.

In some patients, rectal disease, such as rectal fistula, fissure, or perirectal abscess, is the first indication of regional enteritis. This is important in both diagnosis and treatment. The usual surgical procedure for these patients is likely to fail if regional enteritis is present. The operative incision heals poorly and incontinence may develop. Removal of the small intestinal disease is often necessary to cure these patients, and occasionally they will need a temporary colostomy to secure healing of the anal incision. In rare cases when the rectum is actually involved by regional enteritis, the fistula will not heal even with a colostomy, and resection will be necessary.

The diagnosis of severe or progressive enteritis can usually be confirmed by gastrointestinal x-ray study. Of 74 patients who came to surgery because of regional enteritis between June 1958 and June 1963 and who had a preoperative gastrointestinal study, evidence of the small bowel disease was revealed in 97.2 percent.[13] With few exceptions, these patients show an increase in small bowel motility, a segmental distribution of barium in the

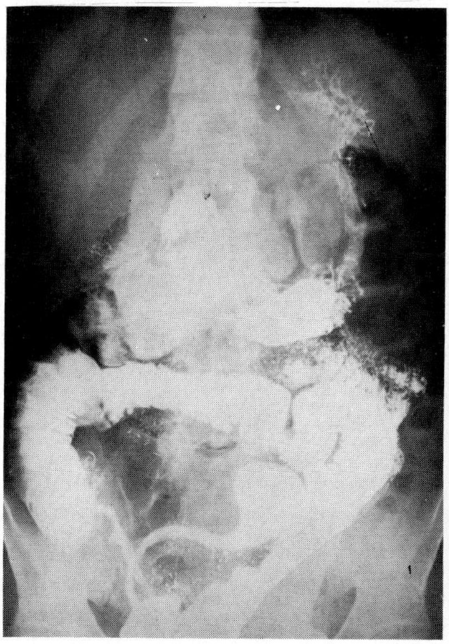

Fig. 5–4.

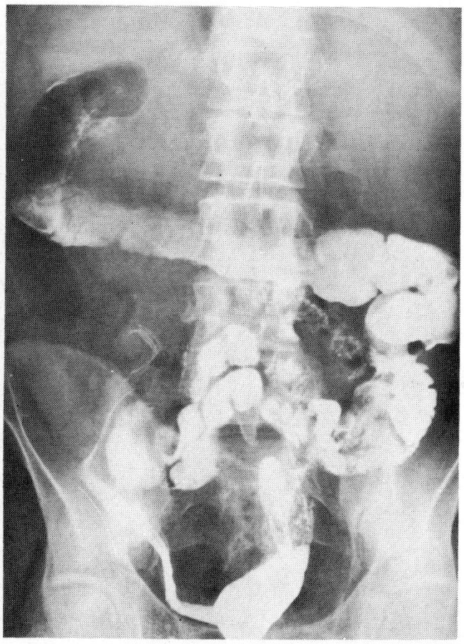

Fig. 5–5.

Figure 5–4. Barium study showing regional enteritis involving terminal ileum. (From Colcock, B. P.: Regional Enteritis. Current Problems in Surgery. Chicago, Year Book Medical Publishers, Inc., 1965, p. 16.)

Figure 5–5. Barium enema illustrating internal fistula between ileum and sigmoid colon. (From Colcock, B. P.: Regional Enteritis. Current Problems in Surgery. Chicago, Year Book Medical Publishers, Inc., 1965, p. 17.)

small bowel, or a markedly narrowed terminal ileum (Fig. 5–4). Hyperirritability of the small bowel with coarsening of the mucosal pattern and evidence of thickening and edema in the intestinal wall are often present.

On the other hand, x-ray examination cannot be relied upon to detect the presence of skip areas or internal fistulas. In our experience, these are rarely discovered before laparotomy.[13] Nine patients were found at operation to have an internal fistula, but this diagnosis was made by preoperative x-ray study in only one patient (Fig. 5–5). In none of the 13 patients with skip areas was the diagnosis made before surgery. Very often the diagnosis is indicated by the finding of enteritis at a previous exploration, or by the presence of an external fistula or mass.

Medical Treatment

Unless acute appendicitis cannot be ruled out, we believe that all patients with regional enteritis should have a trial of medical therapy. The diet is a bland, milk-free, low-residue diet, similar to that for patients who have ulcerative colitis. Antibiotics, usually Chloromycetin or Achromycin, are given if fever is present. These patients need plenty of rest, and this means bed rest in the acute stage. General measures such as the administration of antispasmodics, the relief of stress, and sedation are also employed.

ACTH and the steroid hormones are thought to be of value in the treatment of regional enteritis, particularly in the early inflammatory stage. For this reason, they should be given early rather than late in the course of the disease. If the patient responds to steroid therapy, it should be tapered off and stopped within three to four weeks after symptomatic recovery.

Steroid therapy may not be effective in the chronic relapsing form of the disease. It is rarely effective in the treatment of acute obstruction, and it is of no value to the patient who has a perforation or a fistula. Despite this fact, most patients with regional enteritis at the present time are given a regimen of steroid therapy or have been given it in the past. This is important because it indicates the need for replacement therapy during the early postoperative period. If steroids have been given for a long time, the intraabdominal disease is likely to be much more extensive than the symptoms would indicate. The technical hazards of the surgical procedure are increased, and the bowel must be handled with extreme care to avoid a perforation and extensive contamination of the peritoneal cavity.

Medical treatment after operation is also indicated for all patients with regional enteritis. They are kept on a bland, low-residue, milk-free diet; adequate rest and general hygienic measures are continued.

SURGICAL TREATMENT

Indications for Surgery

Most patients who have regional enteritis require operation either because their symptoms have not responded to medical treatment, or because one of the complications of the disease has developed. The most common

Table 5-1. Principal Indications for Operation (85 Patients)*

SYMPTOMS	NO. OF PATIENTS
Small bowel obstruction	40 (47%)
Severe diarrhea	11
Abdominal mass	10
Severe pain	8
Enterocutaneous fistula	6
Perforation	5
Bladder fistula	2
Abscess	1
Loss of weight	1
Bleeding	1

* From Colcock, B. P., and Fortin, C.: Ann. Surg. *161:*813 (May) 1965.

complication is obstruction of the small intestine. The attacks of cramplike abdominal pain become more frequent and more severe. The patient is unwilling to eat because it increases his pain, so he becomes malnourished and anemic.

A tender abdominal mass often develops, usually in the right lower abdominal quadrant. If the mass is fixed and adherent to the abdominal wall, it usually indicates a perforation with the formation of an abscess. This in turn may lead to an internal or an enterocutaneous fistula. Other patients require surgical intervention because of a steady deterioration in their general condition as a result of intractable diarrhea. The principal indications for surgery in the 85 patients operated on between June 1958 and June 1963 are listed in Table 5–1.[13]

Preparation

Patients with regional enteritis require careful preparation for surgery, since they are likely to be malnourished and anemic. Secondary infection is combated with antibiotics and the anemia is corrected with blood transfusions. Rest in bed, a bland, low-residue diet, and antispasmodics may help the intractable diarrhea, but operation should not be delayed too long if they do not start to improve. This is particularly true if the patient has small bowel obstruction. A long intestinal tube may be passed into the small intestine for decompression, but only surgery will permanently relieve the small bowel obstruction.

Technique

In a number of patients, regional enteritis is discovered at the time of laparotomy for acute appendicitis or other intraabdominal disease. The procedure employed depends upon the extent of the disease and the associated operative conditions. If diffuse peritonitis is present, it is hazardous to carry out definitive therapy. The abdomen may be closed, and some patients may have no further trouble from their regional enteritis. In many, however, persistent or recurrent symptoms develop. When the acute process has subsided and the disease has progressed to the chronic cicatricial stage (usually producing obstruction), resection can be done with very little risk.

If the surgeon encounters a localized acute inflammatory process involving the terminal ileum and cecum, it is often possible to exteriorize the entire mass along with the ascending colon and terminal ileum. Resection and anastomosis can then be performed without contamination of the peritoneal cavity, and since the proximal ileum and colon are normal, they can be anastomosed with safety.

When a significant degree of small bowel obstruction is encountered, this must be corrected even though peritonitis is present. The procedure employed depends upon the extent of the inflammatory reaction and the condition of the proximal ileum. A side-to-side ileocolostomy between the ileum and transverse colon may be carried out, or the proximal ileum can be exteriorized as an ileostomy and the distal segment as a mucous fistula. Resection of the involved bowel with anastomosis can be performed later.

If the surgeon decides to close the abdomen or to carry out a bypass procedure, the question arises: Should an appendectomy be done? We know that removal of the appendix in the presence of regional enteritis often leads to an enterocutaneous fistula. The fistula may arise from the diseased bowel rather than the appendiceal stump, but the result is the same: it will not heal. Twenty-five percent of our patients with an enterocutaneous fistula have had a recent appendectomy. On the other hand, if the surgeon does not remove the appendix in these patients, a potentially dangerous situation is created. Subsequent symptoms such as pain or tenderness in the right lower quadrant are likely to be attributed to recurrent enteritis, and appendectomy will not be performed. This could result in a tragedy if the patient actually has acute appendicitis.

Since he cannot rule out acute appendicitis, the surgeon may decide to operate, only to find that the symptoms were, indeed, the result of recurrence of the regional enteritis. He is then faced with an awkward, although less vital, decision. He can close the abdomen; he can remove a normal appendix; or he can resect the recurrent disease, knowing that it might subside with conservative treatment. These problems would arise less frequently if the appendix were removed whenever it appeared safe to do so. We remove the appendix unless the inflammatory process involves the cecal wall. Removal of the appendix with careful inversion of the stump is not likely to lead to a fistula if the wall of the cecum is not involved by enteritis. If the cecal wall is involved by extension of the inflammatory process from the terminal ileum, the appendix is left alone. Since a persistent ileocutaneous fistula often arises from the diseased terminal ileum rather than the appendiceal stump, the surgeon should not disturb the inflammatory process if he does not intend to resect it.

For many years, one of the most controversial questions regarding the surgical treatment of regional enteritis has been whether the treatment of choice for these patients should be a bypass procedure or a resection. We have always preferred resection, but under certain circumstances, a bypass may be the procedure of choice. In the older patient, symptoms of regional enteritis may be caused by a chronic, stenotic contracture of the terminal ileum associated with very little acute inflammation. If the surgeon is concerned about the ability of such a patient to withstand resection, he can bypass the obstruction with a side-to-side anastomosis between the ileum and transverse colon. This will relieve the patient of his symptoms with very little risk, and he may have no further symptoms (Fig. 5–6).

In other patients with an acute inflammatory process, the dilatation and edema of the proximal small bowel may be so great that resection and anastomosis would be hazardous. A side-to-side anastomosis between the

Figure 5–6. Ileotransverse colostomy for cicatricial stenosis of terminal ileum due to regional enteritis. (From Colcock, B. P.: Regional Enteritis. Current Problems in Surgery. Chicago, Year Book Medical Publishers, Inc., 1965, p. 29.)

Figure 5–7. Ileotransverse colostomy with exclusion. (From Colcock, B. P.: Regional Enteritis. Current Problems in Surgery. Chicago, Year Book Medical Publishers, Inc., 1965, p. 29.)

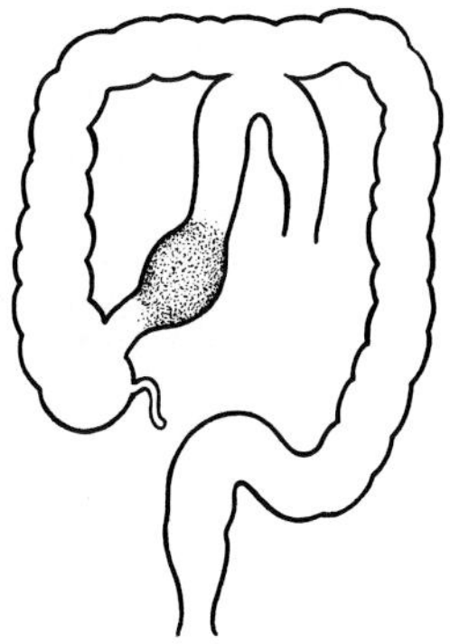

Fig. 5–6.

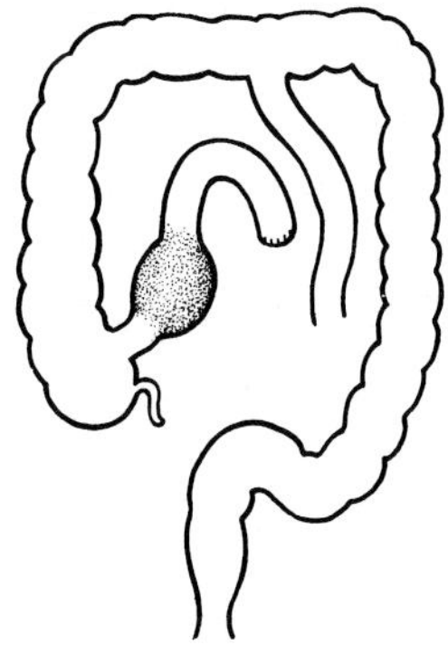

Fig. 5–7.

ileum and transverse colon can be done as the first stage of a two-stage procedure. If symptoms persist or recur, the disease process in the bypassed segment may be resected later. By that time, the dilatation of the small bowel will have disappeared and its distal end can be closed securely. Two-stage procedures, however, are rarely necessary in the surgical treatment of regional enteritis.

Barber et al.[2] and Stahlgren and Ferguson[49] also believe that resection of the diseased bowel is the procedure of choice. Bypass procedures are reserved for patients in the acutely obstructed phase of the disease and for those with extensive disease.

Surgeons who have had the most experience with the bypass procedure maintain that it should be done by the exclusion method if the best result is to be obtained (Fig. 5–7). The small bowel above the diseased segment is divided, the upper end is anastomosed to the transverse colon, and the distal end is closed. This excludes the involved segment from the fecal stream and should result in more rapid resolution of the inflammatory process. A word of caution is in order regarding this procedure. If the enteritis has narrowed the bowel lumen almost to the point of obstruction, closure of the bowel above the disease creates a closed loop. That such a situation is more than a theoretical hazard is indicated by the fact that dilatation and leakage from this closed loop have occurred with very serious results.

We believe that removal of the chronically infected bowel and mesentery gives the patient with regional enteritis his best chance to get well quickly and to remain well (Fig. 5–8). Today there is fairly general agreement that resection is the procedure of choice. First, the inflammatory process does not always subside when it is bypassed, even by the exclusion method. We have operated on many patients several months after a short-circuiting procedure had been performed only to find extensive acute inflammation, including small abscesses, still present in the bowel wall and mesentery. When one considers the marked tendency of this disease to persist or to recur, it does not seem advisable to leave this extensive inflammatory

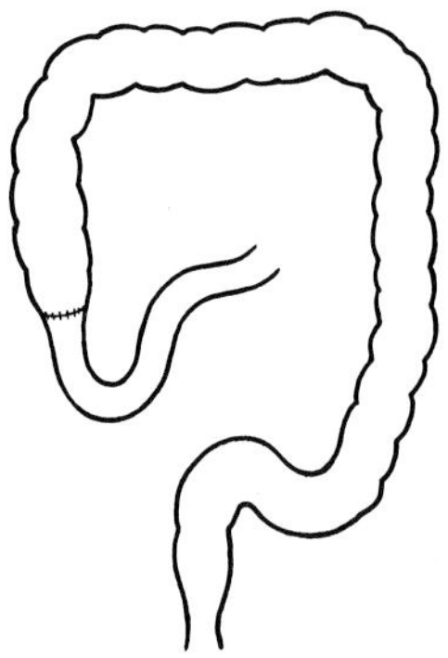

Figure 5–8. Resection and anastomosis. (From Colcock, B. P.: Regional Enteritis. Current Problems in Surgery. Chicago, Year Book Medical Publishers, Inc., 1965, p. 32.)

process within the abdomen to be absorbed by the patient. Second, the mortality rate for resection is now as low as it is for the bypass procedure. This eliminates what was once considered the main advantage of the more conservative operation. The patient gains nothing from preserving this excluded bypassed bowel, since it no longer takes part in the absorption of fluid and nourishment. Indeed, unless dissection of the inflammatory process is carried out, a much longer segment of small bowel may be bypassed than is actually involved by the regional enteritis. Many times adjacent loops of bowel become adherent to the inflammatory process, but are essentially normal as far as function is concerned. Third, our experience in the use of a bypass procedure has not been favorable. Of the 304 patients with regional enteritis who were reported in 1960, 30 patients were treated by a short-circuiting procedure.[14] Sixteen of these patients subsequently required resection. Recurrent symptoms developed in 10, but were controlled by medical therapy. Of the 85 patients who have been operated on since that report, 5 who had initial bypass procedures have already required resection for persistent or recurrent disease.[13]

The amount of bowel to be resected depends upon the extent of the disease. If the enteritis involves the terminal ileum, the right colon as well as the terminal ileum is mobilized and brought outside the abdomen. This will permit resection and anastomosis of the uninvolved ileum to the colon with no danger of contamination of the peritoneal cavity. Since experience has shown that recurrent disease rarely involves the colon, it is advisable to conserve as much large bowel as possible. For this reason, we long ago stopped doing a routine right colectomy for patients with regional enteritis involving the terminal ileum. A margin of 5 to 7 cm. distal to the disease is sufficient. This usually means removal of only the cecum. Although the cecum and ascending colon have a relatively thin wall and were formerly considered to be unsuitable for anastomosis, leakage from the suture line has not occurred. If there is normal ileum distal to the disease, this may also be conserved. Preservation of as much water-absorbing bowel as possible helps to prevent diarrhea postoperatively. It is difficult, however, to determine just where the disease begins and ends in the small intestine. Since recurrence develops just proximal to the anastomosis, it is well to remove an adequate margin of normal small bowel above the obviously diseased segment. If desired, a frozen section examination of the margin may be made.

Approximately 15 percent of our patients have skip areas of enteritis involving the proximal ileum or jejunum in addition to the disease in the terminal ileum. The decision for or against resection of these skip areas depends upon the severity of the disease. If the skip areas are numerous but are not associated with marked thickening and obstruction of the small bowel, they are usually not removed. We know from experience that in many patients who require a second operation, the disease producing the symptoms is just proximal to the suture line, and the skip areas found at the first procedure show no significant change. On the other hand, if a second segment of ileum or jejunum shows thickening with signs of obstruction, it should be resected. If a long segment of apparently normal bowel is present between the two areas of involvement, it can be conserved by doing two segmental resections.

The greatly enlarged lymph nodes in the mesentery are a characteristic feature of regional enteritis. The value of removing these nodes has never been definitely determined. Since the disease is thought by some to arise in the lymphatics of the small bowel mesentery, it may be that these large infected nodes constitute a source of recurrent disease. It is well known that recurrence is more frequent in patients with this type of involvement.[49] On the other hand, it has not yet been proved that the disease begins in the lymphatics of the small bowel mesentery or that these chronically infected glands contain the primary etiologic agent. They could be simply a response to long-standing suppuration in an extensive disease process. To remove all palpably enlarged nodes completely would often mean the sacrifice of a considerable amount of normal small bowel because its blood supply would have to be divided. At the present time our policy is to remove as many of these nodes as possible without sacrificing the blood supply to the uninvolved intestine. Since we do not know in which patient a recurrence will develop, it is advisable to conserve as much normal bowel as possible in every patient.

The anastomosis can be carried out by any one of the standard methods. Our preference is for an end-to-end anastomosis between the ileum and the colon (Fig. 5–9). Any disparity in the size of the lumen of the large and small intestine is easily corrected by dividing the small bowel obliquely and keeping the disparity in mind as the sutures are placed. Because many of these patients have some degree of obstruction, the lumen of the small bowel is often just as large as that of the colon.

We prefer interrupted sutures for both the inner and outer rows. Although a moderate degree of narrowing at the anastomosis will do no harm because of the semiliquid nature of the small bowel contents, it is desirable to have as large a lumen as possible. It is possible that stasis at the anasto-

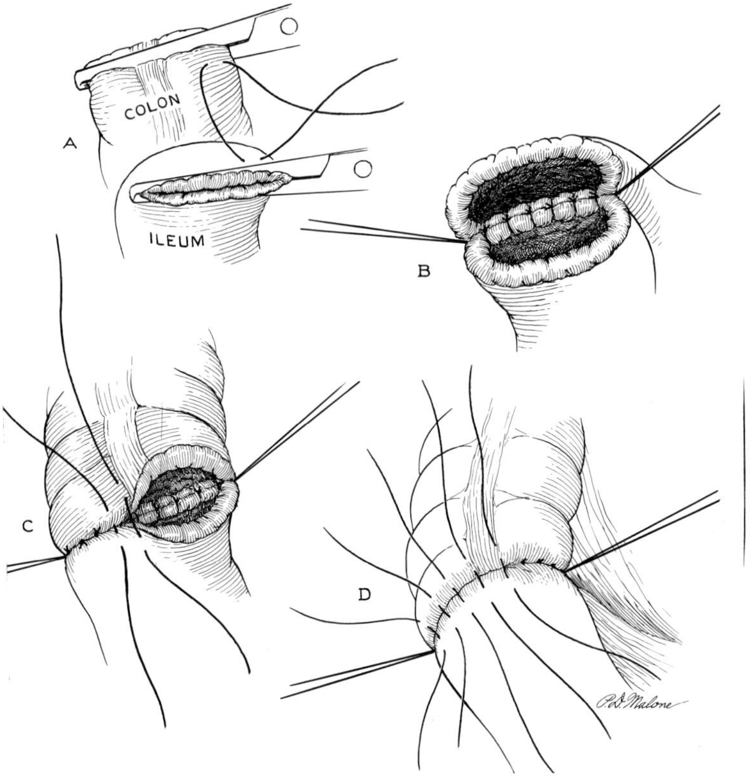

Figure 5–9. Technique of end-to-end anastomosis.

mosis might be a factor in the development of recurrent disease. The inner row of sutures may be of either silk or catgut and are through-and-through sutures, catching the tough submucosa. The outer row is of silk and is placed so as to produce serosa-to-serosa apposition completely around the circumference of the anastomosis. The suture at each end of the anastomosis and in the middle is tied and held. This facilitates the introduction of the remaining sutures in each of the four quadrants.

When the anastomosis has been completed, the opening in the mesentery between the large and small intestine is closed by a running catgut suture, carefully avoiding the blood supply to the bowel. The right lumbar gutter is then reperitonealized. Occasionally, it may be necessary to use the omentum to cover all of the raw surface. As a rule, drainage is not employed, and the right paramedian incision is closed in layers. These patients are usually young, and wound disruption is rare.

A special problem arises when regional enteritis involves the duodenum and produces obstruction (Fig. 5–10). A posterior gastroenterostomy is the procedure of choice in this situation unless active bleeding is present. It is

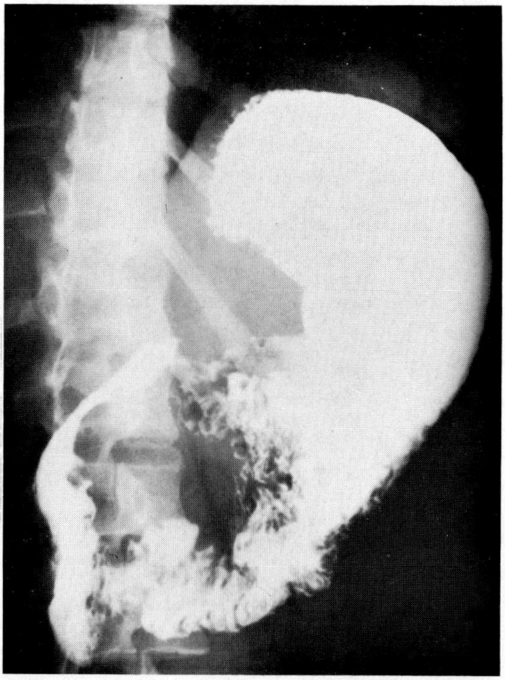

Figure 5–10. Regional enteritis involving the duodenum. (From Colcock, B. P.: Current Problems in Surgery. Chicago, Year Book Medical Publishers, Inc., 1965, p. 34.)

well to add a vagotomy. We have recently operated on a patient for a jejunal ulcer at the site of a gastrojejunostomy carried out several years before for regional enteritis of the duodenum. Rarely, severe hemorrhage develops when the duodenum is involved. In such instances, the disease must be resected to prevent exsanguination. The best approach to this segment of the small bowel is to divide the posterior parietal attachment of the small bowel mesentery completely. The ileum, jejunum, and ascending colon can then be elevated out of the wound and temporarily placed on the patient's chest. This procedure provides an excellent exposure of the second and third portions of the duodenum, and resection can be carried out without serious difficulty.[11] Rarely also, subtotal gastrectomy will be necessary for pyloric obstruction resulting from regional enteritis.

Recently, there has been a tendency to divide regional enteritis clinically into the acute and chronic phases. Since this may have a direct bearing upon its clinical management, it is worth considering. The unknown factor is the number of cases in which the disease first manifests itself in the acute form, but is simply an acute exacerbation of a long-standing unrecognized process. Until ulceration occurs, regional enteritis rarely causes sufficient symptoms to justify exploratory operation.

In a review of 75 patients seen at the Vancouver General Hospital, MacKenzie and colleagues[35] found that in the 20 cases of acute enteritis: (1) the enteritis was confined to the terminal ileum, (2) the symptoms simulated those of acute appendicitis, (3) fistula did not develop after an appendectomy in 17 cases, and (4) only one patient returned with the chronic form of the disease.

In the 55 cases of chronic enteritis, they found that the duration of symptoms averaged 32 months. The most common symptoms were pain and diarrhea—and bleeding if the colon was involved. A mass was present in 38 percent, and anorectal lesions were found in 18 percent. The recurrence rate was 38 percent and the reoperative rate was 30 percent. Resection was the treatment of choice, and there was no operative mortality.

In a recent review of 42 cases of "acute" regional enteritis, Crohn[18] stated that nearly half recovered without resection after conservative treatment with broad-spectrum antibiotics. In the others, he thought the passage of time reduced the risk of the eventual surgery required for chronic granulomatous ileitis.

Complications

Serious postoperative complications are not common following resection for regional enteritis. An occasional abdominal abscess will require incision and drainage; a leak from the anastomosis may give rise to an enterocutaneous fistula. Since the disease has been removed and there is no obstruction distal to the anastomosis, these fistulas heal spontaneously.

If a large amount of ileum has been removed, these patients may require medication to control diarrhea because of the loss of water-absorbing intestine. In patients who have had extensive resections of the small bowel, symptoms suggesting the malabsorption syndrome may develop. They may have weight loss, hypoproteinemia, hypocalcemia, hypokalemia, osteoporosis, and severe anemia. The management of this short bowel malabsorption syndrome is considered in Chapter Six.

Mortality Rate

The mortality rate for the surgical treatment of regional enteritis is low, even though almost all these patients have had a resection of the disease. Of 346 resections carried out for regional enteritis prior to June 1958, the operative mortality rate was 1.7 percent.[14] One death occurred among 85 patients who have been operated on since that time.[13] This was the first operative death since 1952, and it occurred in a patient who had both ulcerative colitis and regional enteritis. This patient had had a complete colectomy for ulcerative colitis and a total of 12 operative procedures for regional enteritis. Despite intensive supportive treatment, most of which was for the relief of recurrent enterocutaneous fistulas, almost all of the anterior abdominal wall was eventually digested away and she finally died. Another patient died several months after discharge from the hospital. This patient, too, had had an ileostomy and colectomy for ulcerative colitis in addition to surgery for regional enteritis.

Recurrence

All these patients are given a bland, low-residue, high-protein diet following operation. If symptoms develop that suggest recurrent disease, these measures are intensified and the patient is given a trial of steroid therapy. A careful follow-up provides an opportunity for recognizing the early stages of the disease, such as edema, beginning ulceration of the mucosa, and so forth. A diagnosis of recurrent disease can usually be established by x-ray examination (Fig. 5–11). (The resected specimen is shown in Figure 5–12.) The mere presence of diarrhea, however, does not necessarily mean recurrent disease.

In our experience, based on follow-up studies of from 5 to 15 years, the recurrence rate is approximately 30 to 35 percent.[13] Twenty-five percent of our patients have required reoperation. It has often been said that the usual proportion of patients who require reoperation is higher than this, yet Barber et al.[2] reported a comparable series of 257 patients in whom only 17 percent required a second operation, and all these patients had follow-up studies for five years. Ninety-three percent of their patients had a primary resection.

Even those patients who have required reoperation have a reasonable chance for cure. In the series, reported by Barber et al.,[2] of 49 patients who

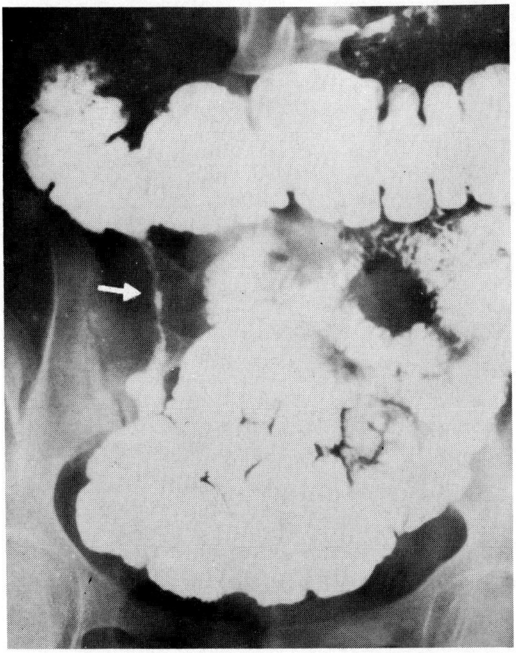

Figure 5–11. Recurrent regional enteritis at and proximal to anastomosis. (From Colcock, B. P.: Regional Enteritis. Chicago, Year Book Medical Publishers, Inc., 1965, p. 31.)

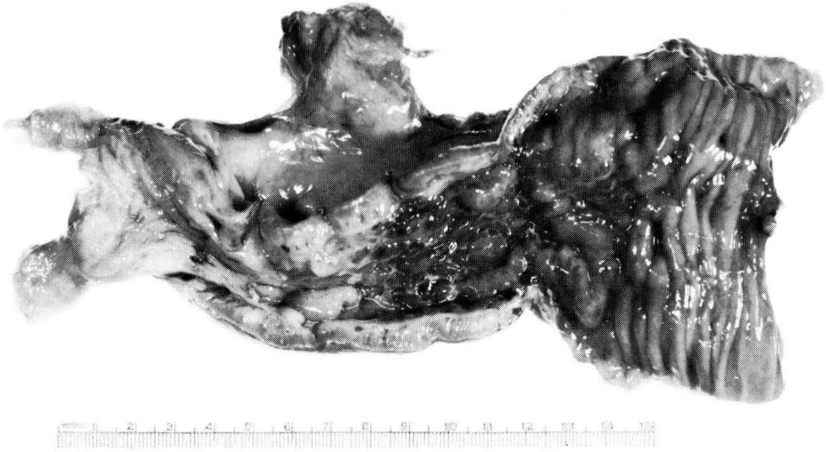

Figure 5–12. Resected specimen from same patient as shown in Figure 5–11.

required an operative procedure because of recurrence, only 15 (30 percent) underwent a third procedure and only 4 of these 15 patients needed a fourth procedure. Our experience has been similar. More than 50 percent of our patients who required a second operation were completely relieved by that procedure, and 50 percent of those who required a third procedure were relieved of their symptoms.

The surgical treatment of patients with regional enteritis is often frustrating, but it is rarely hopeless. One must keep in mind that patients with regional enteritis do not come to surgery for their first, their second or their third operation unless intensive medical treatment has failed. They have no one to turn to except the surgeon. We agree with Barber et al.[2] and with Stahlgren and Ferguson[49] that more than 75 percent of patients who have persistent or recurrent regional enteritis will be rehabilitated by a combination of surgical and medical treatment.

SUMMARY

Regional enteritis is a disease of unknown etiology with no specific medical treatment. Many patients who have this disease require surgical intervention because of obstruction, perforation, or the development of a fistula. The treatment of choice is resection of the disease. The surgical mortality rate is low and postoperative complications are few. The recurrence rate, however, remains high. Twenty-five percent of these patients will require reoperation because of a recurrence that cannot be controlled by medical management. Nevertheless, the great majority of these patients can be restored to reasonably good health by a combination of surgical and medical therapy.

TUBERCULOSIS

With the advent of chemotherapy of pulmonary and other forms of tuberculosis, the incidence of intestinal tuberculosis has been greatly reduced. Tuberculosis of the intestine is caused most commonly by the human strain of the organism that has been ingested. The organism lodges most commonly in areas of stasis, regions with abundant lymphoid tissue, and areas of increased rate of absorption.[29, 47] Thus, in decreasing order of frequency, the infection is found in the ileum, colon, jejunum, appendix, sigmoid colon, rectum, duodenum, stomach, and esophagus (Table 5–2).[48] Approximately 85 percent of the lesions are in the ileocecal area and most are secondary to pulmonary involvement.

In the area of predilection, the bacillus becomes localized in the depths of the mucosal glands. It is carried from there by the lymphatics to the Peyer's patches.[44] Here, as a result of inflammation, sloughing of tissue, and local attempts at healing and walling off, the three typical appearances of the disease become evident. These are the ulcerative, hypertrophic, or ulcero-hypertrophic types.

The gross picture of the disease may show submucosal edema, cellular infiltration, ulcerations, tubercle formation visible on the serosal surface, lymphadenopathy with or without caseation, and fibrosis of the bowel wall with enormous thickening of the mesentery.

The histologic diagnosis of the disease may be difficult and is based on the findings of caseating tubercles and acid-fast tubercle bacilli.[8, 40] The demonstration of the tubercle bacillus on culture or guinea pig inoculation is helpful. After antituberculous chemotherapy, these findings may be obscured and great difficulty may be encountered in differentiating this disease from regional enteritis.

Tuberculosis of the gastrointestinal tract has in the past been seen predominantly in young adults, being more prevalent in females. It occurs in autopsy series in from 51 to 70 percent of patients with pulmonary tuberculosis.[20, 52] Blumberg[7] reported the roentgenographic incidence to be

Table 5–2. Sites of Involvement of Tuberculosis of the Gastrointestinal Tract in Decreasing Frequency*

MORE FREQUENT	LESS FREQUENT
Ileum	Rectum
Colon	Duodenum
Jejunum	Stomach
Appendix	Esophagus

* Adapted from Riggins, H. M.: M. Clin. North America *26*:823 (May) 1942.

Table 5–3. Symptoms of Gastrointestinal Tuberculosis*

	PERCENT
Abdominal pain	60
Weight loss	59
Nausea	44
Diarrhea	18

* Adapted from Bockus, H. L.: Gastroenterology. Ed. 2. Philadelphia, W. B. Saunders Co., 1964, p. 317.

5 to 8 percent in patients with early pulmonary disease. These statistics are based on studies of patients before the antibiotic era and are not valid for current practice.

Gastrointestinal tuberculosis is varied in its manifestations. Abdominal pain (60 percent), weight loss (59 percent), nausea (44 percent), and diarrhea (18 percent) are suggestive of intestinal involvement (Table 5–3).[8] Most commonly, the majority of patients (71 percent) with radiographic evidence of intestinal tuberculosis have no symptoms or signs of the disease.[32] This complication of pulmonary tuberculosis should be considered when: (1) lung cavitation is present with a highly positive sputum; (2) abdominal symptoms appear, not having been present previously; (3) sudden reversal of a previously satisfactory clinical course occurs unexplained by alteration in the pulmonary status; and (4) the clinical course does not respond to adequate treatment.

The findings on physical examination are apt to be minimal. At times, a tender, fixed mass can be palpated in the right lower quadrant. With the development of complications, the findings are those of the complications.

Radiographic examination demonstrates changes reflecting the stage of the pathologic process. Irritability of the involved loop leads to nonfilling of that loop. Hypertrophy, edema, and overgrowth of tissue lead to obstruction. As with all granulomatous lesions of the cecum, filling defects may be seen in this area.

The complications of intestinal tuberculosis include obstruction, free perforation into the peritoneal cavity, abscess or fistula, hemorrhage, intussusception, and the formation of traction diverticula. One autopsy series revealed an incidence of these complications of 23 percent.[34] The systemic complications of this disease are frequent and include malnutrition and amyloidosis.

Tuberculous peritonitis is a particularly grave complication.[24] The entire abdomen is usually tender, occasionally rigid, and may contain masses. The typical doughy abdomen is found in only 10 percent or less of cases. There may be a rapid onset of this complication with pain, chills, and fever. Ascites is frequent. The white blood cell count is usually normal.

The primary treatment of enteric tuberculosis is based on the use of antituberculous drugs and measures to increase the patient's resistance to the infection. Combinations of isoniazid, streptomycin, and para-aminosalicylate are preferred. Rest, and a bland, low-residue diet (low in fat if diarrhea is present) are important.

Surgical therapy is usually limited to the treatment of the complications. These include perforation, obstruction, and hemorrhage. However, there is some indication for the surgical treatment of uncomplicated hypertrophic disease since this form does not respond to drug therapy as well as other forms.[1] At times, surgical resection of the diseased intestine is the only method available for determining the diagnosis, especially in primary tuberculous enteritis. In fact, Faulkner[24] reported that surgical treatment in his series was initiated usually because of an undiagnosed mass or radiographic shadow.

The general principles of surgical therapy in this condition have not been clearly redefined since the advent of chemotherapy. However, it seems likely that tuberculous peritonitis is not a surgical disease.[24] If operative treatment is chosen, the tuberculous lesion is resected when feasible, and the majority of these patients have excellent results.[1, 24, 51] Bypass procedures and simple closure and drainage of perforations are often followed by recurring complications, fistulas, and death.[24, 51] When the cecum is to be resected, the terminal ileum should be included in the resection, and vice versa, since 80 to 90 percent of lesions involving either section of intestine indeed involve both.[1]

If the diagnosis of tuberculous enteritis is known or suspected preoperatively, and if the contemplated operative procedure is elective, an antituberculous chemotherapy program of one or two weeks should be carried out preoperatively.[1] This preparation includes daily administration of isoniazid, 300 mg., and aminosalicylic acid, 12 gm. Streptomycin is given in a dose of 1 gm. the day preceding surgery and daily for one week postoperatively. Isoniazid and aminosalicylic acid therapy are continued for 6 to 12 months postoperatively.

The results of antituberculous treatment for uncomplicated intestinal disease are generally good if the patient can be kept under observation.[37] Most often a successful result with the intestinal phase of the disease is predicated on a successful result with the pulmonary involvement.

Rarely, intestinal tuberculosis is secondary to pelvic infection, or it may occur primarily in this location.[47] In these instances the bovine strain is usually responsible;[6] however, Ukil,[52] working in India, recovered the human strain in the majority of his cases. The pathologic type of lesion is usually hypertrophic.[8, 40] The symptoms, diagnosis, and treatment of this variant are similar to the usual secondary disease.

TYPHOID ENTERITIS

Typhoid fever, an acute illness caused by Salmonella typhi, is a disease capable of causing ulceration, with hemorrhage or perforation of the small intestine.[4, 30, 50] Infection is by the oral route, from contaminated food or drink. The organism lodges in the lymphoid tissue of the wall of the small intestine (Peyer's patches) and moves from there to the mesenteric nodes, liver, and general circulation.

The clinical manifestations may vary from none when the patient is in the carrier state to a fulminating process that overwhelms the patient within a few days. A case of average severity may last six to eight weeks after an average 10-day to 12-day incubation period when malaise, headache, and fever are noted. There also may be generalized abdominal discomfort. By the third week the temperature varies between 102° and 104° F. daily. With the high fever, diarrhea may commence. After a period of fever lasting one to two weeks, the disease gradually subsides. The average duration of illness is about 30 days for the untreated case.

The physical signs include splenomegaly in the second week. A rash (rose spots) is seen during the second or third week and appears characteristically on the trunk. At the height of the illness, generalized abdominal tenderness and distention are seen.

Normochromic anemia and leukopenia are usually present. The feces are usually positive for occult blood during the third and fourth weeks of illness, and sometimes gross blood is seen. In the early weeks the blood cultures may be positive for Salmonella typhi, and by the third or fourth week of the illness the stool cultures are usually positive. Demonstration of a positive Widal reaction is strong evidence for the diagnosis of typhoid fever.

Hemorrhage, perforation, and acute cholecystitis are the important abdominal complications. The intestinal complications are the result of ulceration and erosion of blood vessels in Peyer's patches. Gross bleeding is present in 10 to 20 percent of all cases, but perforation occurs in only about 2 percent of cases.

The treatment of typhoid fever is chloramphenicol, which is specific for the disease.[58] Doses of 3 to 4 gm. a day are continued until the fever abates—usually three days. Thereafter 1 to 2 gm. a day is given for one and one half to two weeks. The patients should be isolated, all attendants immunized, and supportive measures instituted. Cortisone, 200 mg. a day, does much to reduce toxicity.[58] Laparotomy is advised for massive uncontrolled bleeding although every effort to avoid operation should be made, as the bleeding is usually from multiple points.[30]

Huckstep[30] advised conservative treatment of perforation, since the involved bowel is exceedingly friable and the results following laparotomy have been disastrous. He advised an operative approach only in cases of sudden perforation in an otherwise good risk, convalescent patient who is seen within six hours of the perforation. He would also perform laparotomy in patients with certain complications of perforation, such as adhesive obstruction or abscess.

Acute typhoid cholecystitis should also be treated conservatively unless empyema makes surgical intervention imperative.[30]

The treatment of the carrier state is beyond the scope of this monograph; however, cholecystectomy should eradicate the intestinal carrier state in about 90 percent of cases when combined with antibiotic therapy.

With ideal treatment, the fatality rate in cases of typhoid fever should be less than 5 percent.

MISCELLANEOUS ENTERITIS

Necrotizing Jejunitis

There is a group of cases of enteritis that are not regional enteritis or bacterial enteritis because of differences in their pathologic appearance and their clinical course. Necrotizing jejunitis is one of these, as are primary jejunitis,[31] jejunitis, and ileitis regionalis acuta.[10] The relationship of "phlegmonous jejunitis" to necrotic jejunitis is unknown, but Fick and Wolken[25] consider them to be separate processes.

Fick and Wolken,[25] working in Northern Germany between the years 1944 and 1949, reported a series of cases that they called necrotic or necrotizing jejunitis. Examination of the involved jejunum showed a high degree of inflammation and necrosis, which was discretely localized. Clostridium welchii, type F, was implicated as the offending organism in one laboratory series.[59] Early in the disease the involved serosa was red and resembled a sausage. In later stages, there was necrosis of the mucosa and submucosa with possible perforation. The involvement of the lymph glands has been described as minimal.[25] The clinical course of the disease was often catastrophic and marked by hemorrhage, perforation, obstruction, and extreme toxicity. If the patient survived, scar formation and obstruction might ensue. Another report[16] described two patients who survived after resection, but the mortality ordinarily is high (16 of 18 patients).[25]

Necrotizing Arteriolitis

The association of an ulcerative jejunitis and the arteriolitis of the so-called collagen diseases of lupus erythematosus, rheumatoid arthritis, and polyarteritis has been noted. One report described three cases with involvement of the small intestine with multiple ulcerations and perforations, each of which ended fatally.[26] Presumably, earlier surgical treatment could have altered the outcome.

PSEUDOMEMBRANOUS ENTEROCOLITIS

Pseudomembranous enterocolitis, an inflammatory condition usually of the small or large intestine, or both, and occasionally found in the stomach, has aroused considerable controversy centering around its etiology.[28, 41] As first described by Finney,[27] the involved intestine shows focal areas of necrosis of the mucosa which coalesce and deepen, leading to the formation of a characteristic pseudomembrane. This membrane formation is accompanied by an inflammatory cellular reaction of the bowel wall.[42]

Clinically, the disease may be ushered in by sudden circulatory collapse, which may be preceded by lethargy, weakness, and abdominal pain. Diarrhea and fever usually follow, associated with toxicity, abdominal distention, nausea, and severe dehydration. The intestine may contain up to several liters of dark fluid. The mortality rate in this disease is high; it approaches 100 percent in some series.

The etiology of pseudomembranous enterocolitis is not settled. Heavy metal poisoning, uremia, septicemia, "shock," and corticosteroid therapy have been considered.[5, 28] Other authors insist it is caused by a staphylococcal infection of the intestine and frequently follows antibiotic administration.[47] Emphasis has been placed on its occurrence after major surgical operations,[41, 43] but Kleckner et al.[33] described 14 cases that did not follow operation. To compound the confusion further, Pettet et al.[43] described 45 cases before the antibiotic era and did not consider that the incidence of the disease had increased in the period 1939 to 1952. Marston[36] and McGovern and Goulston[38] who believe that this disease is the result of ischemic necrosis of the bowel mucosa are in the minority.

The treatment of the condition is dependent on the early suspicion of this disease in the prodromal stages of toxicity, irritability, and hypotension. Massive fluid replacement with electrolytes, plasma, and blood are essential. Decompression of the intestinal tract by tube is helpful. The use of vasoconstrictors and corticosteroids has been encouraged by some. An antistaphylococcal drug must also be given.

STAPHYLOCOCCAL ENTEROCOLITIS

The differentiation of idiopathic pseudomembranous enterocolitis from staphylococcal enterocolitis is not clear. Prohaska[45] has reproduced pseudomembranous enterocolitis in antibiotic-treated chinchillas by the oral administration of staphylococci or by the oral administration of staphylococcal enterotoxin. Furthermore, he believed that all cases of pseudomembranous enterocolitis are due to staphylococcus toxin and staphylococcus overgrowth in the bowel.[45, 46] Certainly, many cases of enterocolitis can end fatally and are due to overgrowth of Staphylococcus aureus. Therefore, in any patient in whom this diagnosis is suspected and in whom gram-stain examination of bowel content shows a preponderance of staphylococci, the supportive treatment just suggested and an antibiotic effective against staphylococci must be instituted. If reports on routine culture examination of the stool are awaited, the patient may die before treatment can be effective. Another form of therapy, the use of enemas containing normal feces to suppress the growth of staphylococci, has been suggested and should be considered.[23]

To prevent postoperative or any type of staphylococcal enterocolitis, serious consideration should be given to the discontinuance of the use of antibiotics as a prophylactic measure and in the preparation of the bowel for surgery. It is indeed open to question whether the antibiotic preparation of the bowel preoperatively is effective in lowering postoperative morbidity and mortality.

One must be careful to avoid labeling all cases of diarrhea following antibiotic treatment as pseudomembranous enterocolitis, since cases of very mild diarrhea might be importantly different entities and require different treatment.[21]

REFERENCES

1. Abrams, J. S., and Holden, W. D.: Tuberculosis of the gastrointestinal tract. Arch. Surg. *89:*282–293 (Aug.) 1964.
2. Barber, K. W., Jr., Waugh, J. M., Beahrs, O. H., et al.: Indications for and the results of the surgical treatment of regional enteritis. Ann. Surg. *156:*472–482 (Sept.) 1962.
3. Bargen, J. A.: Discussion. J.A.M.A. *99:*1328 (Oct. 15) 1932.
4. Beeson, P. B., and McDermott, W.: Cecil-Loeb Textbook of Medicine. Ed. 11. Philadelphia, W. B. Saunders Co., 1963, Vol. I, pp. 235–239.
5. Birnbaum, D., Laufer, A., and Freund, M.: Pseudomembranous enterocolitis. A clinicopathologic study. Gastroenterology *41:*345–352 (Oct.) 1961.
6. Blackblock, J. W. S.: Tuberculous diseases in children. Medical Research Council. Spec. Rep. Sev. 172, London. His Majesty's Stationery Office, 1932.
7. Blumberg, A.: Pathology of intestinal tuberculosis. J. Lab. & Clin. Med. *13:*405–412 (Feb.) 1928.
8. Bockus, H. L.: Gastroenterology. Vol. II. The Small Intestine, Absorption and Nutrition; the Colon, Peritoneum, Mesentery and Omentum. Ed. 2. Philadelphia, W. B. Saunders Co., 1964, pp. 311–329.
9. Bockus, H. L.: Gastroenterology. Vol. II. The Small Intestine, Absorption and Nutrition; the Colon, Peritoneum, Mesentery and Omentum. Ed. 2. Philadelphia, W. B. Saunders Co., 1964, p. 231.
10. Brynjulfsen, B. C.: Jejunitis acuta-ileitis regionalis acuta. Acta chir. scandinav. *96:*361–387, 1948.
11. Cattell, R. B., and Braasch, J. W.: A technique for the exposure of the third and fourth portions of the duodenum. Surg. Gynec. & Obst. *111:*378–379 (Sept.) 1960.
12. Colcock, B. P.: Regional Enteritis. Current Problems in Surgery. Chicago, Year Book Medical Publishers, Inc., 1965.
13. Colcock, B. P., and Fortin, C.: Surgical treatment of regional enteritis: Review of 85 cases. Ann. Surg. *161:*812–818 (May) 1965.
14. Colcock, B. P., and Vansant, J. H.: Surgical treatment of regional enteritis. New England J. Med. *262:*435–439 (Mar. 3) 1960.
15. Colcock, B. P., Vansant, J. H., and Contreras, O.: Surgical treatment of coexisting regional enteritis and ulcerative colitis. Surg. Gynec. & Obst. *112:*96–100 (Jan.) 1961.

16. Colman, J. V., and Nield, J. M.: Severe small bowel hemorrhage: necrotizing enteritis. M. J. Australia *1:*355–357 (Mar. 6) 1965.
17. Combe, C., and Saunders, W.: A singular case of stricture and thickening of the ileum; case report presented before Royal College of Physicians in London, July, 1806. Medical Transactions, College of Physicians, London, 1813, Vol. IV, pp. 16–21.
18. Crohn, B. B.: Acute regional ileitis; clinical aspects and follow-up studies. New York J. Med. *65:*641–644 (Mar. 1) 1965.
19. Crohn, B. B., Ginsburg, L., and Oppenheimer, G. D.: Regional ileitis; a pathologic and clinical entity. J.A.M.A. *99:*1323–1329 (Oct. 15) 1932.
20. Cullen, J. H.: Intestinal tuberculosis. A clinical pathological study. Quart. Bull. Sea View Hosp. *5:*143–160 (Jan.) 1940.
21. Cummins, A. J.: Pseudomembranous enterocolitis and the pathology of nosology. Am. J. Digest. Dis. *6:*429–431 (May) 1961.
22. Dalziel, T. K.: Chronic interstitial enteritis. Brit. M. J. *2:*1068–1070 (Oct. 25) 1913.
23. Eiseman, B., Silen, W., Bascom, G. S., et al.: Fecal enema as an adjunct in the treatment of pseudomembranous enterocolitis. Surgery *44:*854–859 (Nov.) 1958.
24. Faulkner, R. L., Jr.: Tuberculosis as a surgical disease of the abdomen. Ann. Surg. *160:*806–813 (Nov.) 1964.
25. Fick, K. A., and Wolken, A. P.: Necrotic jejunitis. Lancet *1:*519–521 (Mar. 26) 1949.
26. Finkbiner, R. B., and Decker, J. P.: Ulceration and perforation of the intestine due to necrotizing arteriolitis. New England J. Med. *268:*14–18 (Jan. 3) 1963.
27. Finney, J. M. T.: Gastro-enterostomy for cicatrizing ulcer of the pylorus. Bull. Johns Hopkins Hosp. *4:*53–55 (May) 1893.
28. Hale, H. W., Jr., and Cosgriff, J. H., Jr.: Pseudomembranous enterocolitis. Am. J. Surg. *94:*710–717 (Nov.) 1957.
29. Hoon, J. R., Dockerty, M. B., and Pemberton, J. deJ.: Collective review; ileocecal tuberculosis including comparison of this disease with nonspecific regional enterocolitis and noncaseous tuberculated enterocolitis. Internat. Abstr. Surg. *60:*417–440, 1950; *in* Surg. Gynec. & Obst. *60* (Nov.) 1950.
30. Huckstep, R. L.: Recent advances in the surgery of typhoid fever. Ann. Roy. Coll. Surgeons England *26:*207–230 (Apr.) 1960.
31. Garner, B. O., Claugus, C. E., and Hamilton, J. E.: Acute perforation of jejunum secondary to primary jejunitis; case report. Ann. Surg. *134:*131–134 (July) 1951.
32. Granet, E.: Intestinal tuberculosis. A clinical, roentgenological and pathological study of 2086 patients affected with pulmonary tuberculosis. Am. J. Digest. Dis. *2:*209–214 (June) 1935.
33. Kleckner, M. S., Jr., Bargen, J. A., and Baggenstoss, A. H.: Pseudomembranous enterocolitis: clinicopathologic study of 14 cases in which disease was not preceded by operation. Gastroenterology *21:*212–222 (June) 1952.
34. Kornblum, S. A., Zale, C., and Aronson, W.: Surgical complications of intestinal tuberculosis as seen at necropsy. Am. J. Surg. *75:*498–501 (Mar.) 1948.
35. MacKenzie, A. D., and colleagues: Personal communication.
36. Marston, A.: The bowel in shock. The role of mesenteric arterial disease as a cause of death in the elderly. Lancet *2:*365–370 (Aug. 25) 1962.
37. Mason, E. F., Kridelbaugh, W. W., Crouch, W. H., et al.: Streptomycin in treatment of tuberculous enteritis; report of 33 cases. Am. J. M. Sc. *217:*28–46 (Jan.) 1949.
38. McGovern, V. J., and Goulston, S. J.: Ischaemic enterocolitis. Gut *6:*213–220 (June) 1965.
39. Meadows, T. R., and Batsakis, J. G.: Histopathological spectrum of regional enteritis. Arch. Surg. *87:*976–981 (Dec.) 1963.
40. Paustian, F. F., and Bockus, H. L.: So-called primary ulcerohypertrophic ileocecal tuberculosis. Am. J. Med. *27:*509–518 (Sept.) 1959.
41. Pearce, C., and Dineen, P.: A study of pseudomembranous enterocolitis. Am. J. Surg. *99:*292–300 (Mar.) 1960.
42. Penner, A., and Bernheim, A. I.: Acute postoperative enterocolitis: A study on the pathologic nature of shock. Arch. Path. *27:*966–983 (June) 1939.
43. Pettet, J. D., Baggenstoss, A. H., Dearing, W. H., et al.: Postoperative pseudomembranous enterocolitis. Surg. Gynec. & Obst. *98:*546–552 (May) 1954.
44. Portis, S. A.: Diseases of the Digestive System. Ed. 3. Philadelphia, Lea & Febiger, 1953.

45. Prohaska, J. V.: Pseudomembranous enterocolitis; the experimental induction of the disease with Staphylococcus aureus and its enterotoxin. Arch. Surg. *79:*197–206 (Aug.) 1959.
46. Prohaska, J. V., Mock, F., Baker, W., et al.: Pseudomembranous (staphylococcal) enterocolitis. Internat. Abstr. Surg. *112:*103–115 (Feb.) 1961; *in* Surg. Gynec. & Obst. *112* (Feb.) 1961.
47. Rankine, J. A.: Tuberculosis of ileocecal area. J. Internat. Coll. Surgeons *18:*202–209 (Aug.) 1952.
48. Riggins, H. M.: Tuberculosis of the alimentary tract. M. Clin. North America *26:*819–829 (May) 1942.
49. Stahlgren, L. H., and Ferguson, L. K.: The results of surgical treatment of chronic regional enteritis. J.A.M.A. *175:*986–989 (Mar. 18) 1961.
50. Stuart, B. M., and Pullen, R. L.: Typhoid; clinical analysis of 360 cases. Arch. Int. Med. *78:*629–661 (Dec.) 1946.
51. Sweetman, W. R., and Wise, R. A.: Acute perforated tuberculous enteritis: surgical treatment. Ann. Surg. *149:*143–148 (Jan.) 1959.
52. Ukil, A. C.: Early diagnosis and treatment of intestinal tuberculosis. Indian M. Gaz. *77:*613–619 (Oct.) 1942.
53. Van Patter, W. N., Bargen, J. A., Dockerty, M. B., et al.: Regional enteritis. Gastroenterology *26:*347–450 (Mar.) 1954.
54. Warren, S., and Sommers, S. C.: Cicatrizing enteritis (regional ileitis) as a pathologic entity; analysis of 120 cases. Am. J. Path. *24:*475–501 (May) 1948.
55. Warren, S., and Sommers, S. C.: Pathogenesis of ulcerative colitis. Am. J. Path. *25:*657–679 (July) 1949.
56. Warren, S., and Sommers, S. C.: Pathology of regional ileitis and ulcerative colitis. J.A.M.A. *154:*189–193 (Jan. 16) 1954.
57. Wilensky, A. O., and Moschcowitz, E.: Non-specific granulomata of intestine. Am. J. Med. Sc. *166:*48–66 (July) 1923.
58. Wisseman, C. L., Jr., et al.: Studies on cortisone and antibiotics for prompt therapeutic control of typhoid fever and scrub typhus. J. Clin. Invest. *33:*264–275 (Feb.) 1954.
59. Zeissler, J., and Rassfeld-Sternberg, L.: Enteritis necroticans due to Clostridium welchii type F. Brit. M. J. *1:*267–269 (Feb. 12) 1949.

Chapter Six

SMALL INTESTINAL INSUFFICIENCY

A distressing and often fatal series of events follows the loss of a critical length of functioning small intestine. The patient with a short bowel suffers from a lack of absorbing surface, and a myriad of deficiencies results. Thus, in the advanced syndrome there is a lack of the majority of the substances absorbed by the small intestine. Since some substances are absorbed in specialized areas of the small intestine, it follows that removal of these areas results in selective deficiency. Selective deficiency also can result from removal of part of the small intestine because of differing efficiencies with which various compounds are absorbed.

BASIC INFORMATION

Normal and Minimal Residual Lengths of Small Intestine

The following points are pertinent as background for any discussion of small bowel insufficiency. The length of the small intestine cannot be measured with accuracy because of its flexibility and because of its pleated mesenteric attachment. The mean length of the mesenteric small bowel (jejunum and ileum) when removed from its mesenteric attachment, has been estimated at approximately 22 feet with a range of from 15 to 33 feet.[30, 65] When the small bowel is measured in situ, its length has been estimated at from 9 to 11 feet.[4] Surveys of collected cases of massive resection indicate that the patient can maintain normal absorptive patterns and weight if at least 50 percent of the small intestine remains and is normal.[10, 30, 40] A remnant of about one third of the small bowel is compatible with life, but with only

Table 6–1. Selected Case Reports Concerning Nutrition and Survival After Massive Small Intestinal Resection

Author and year	Remaining mesenteric small bowel	Observation period	Result
Kinney et al.[38] 1962	None	13 mo.	Death
Althausen et al.[2] 1949	6″ jejunum	1 yr.	3–6 soft foul stools per day; malnutrition and extreme morbidity; wt. 140 to 88 lb.
Wilkie[69] 1950	6″ jejunum	1½ yr.	Deficiencies and psychosis; wt. 135 to 90 lb.
Weckesser[67] 1949	1′ jejunum	10 mo.	Anemia, starvation; death; wt. 127 to 88 lb.
Meyer[51] 1962	1½′ jejunum	16 yr.	Well and working; wt. 145 to 124 lb.
Coleman and Bennett[14] 1942	2½′ jejunum	2 yr.	Heavy work as fisherman; wt. 140 to 90 to 117 lb.
Booth[9] 1961	2½′ jejunum	2½ yr.	Infant; gained wt. normally; macrocytic anemia treated
West et al.[68] 1938	1′ jejunum 2′ ileum	4 yr.	Low calcium tetany; light work
Croot[15] 1952	4–5′ jejunum	10 yr.	Complete recovery; wt. 130 to 85 lb., then gained unknown amount; developed peptic ulcer

this length of functioning bowel present, severe deficiencies can be expected,[10] and survival is not always certain.[30, 32] Although short-term survival has been reported with very short remnants of small intestine,[19, 38, 49, 50] long-term survival is unusual.[42] At least 1 or 2 feet of mesenteric intestine appears necessary to maintain life, although 3 or 4 feet is probably minimal for reasonable health (Table 6–1).

SITES AND EFFICIENCY OF ABSORPTION

Information relative to the site and mechanism of absorption of carbohydrate, fat, protein, water, minerals, electrolytes, and vitamins is not complete (see Chapter Two). Our present knowledge is summarized in Figure 6–1. Both the jejunum and ileum are capable of absorbing all these substances with the exception of vitamin B_{12} and bile salts, which are absorbed exclusively in the ileum. Water absorption is likewise maximal in the ileum and right colon. Of the three foodstuffs, carbohydrate absorption is most complete and is accomplished in the shortest length of intestine. Amino acid absorption is usually complete by the time the chyme reaches the ileum. Fat presents the absorbing mechanism with its greatest problem in

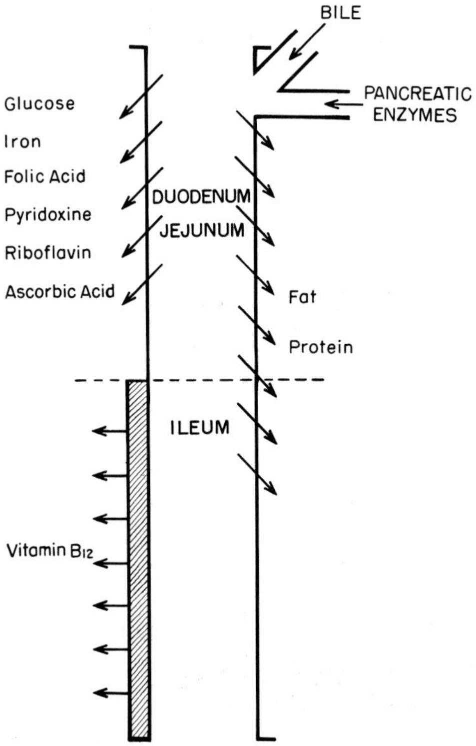

Figure 6–1. Sites of absorption of various substances in normal small intestine.

that it is least efficiently absorbed. There is almost always some spillover of ingested fat from the jejunum into the ileum. Information concerning the relative ability of the jejunum and ileum to absorb fat is controversial.[9] The studies of Kremen et al.[41] and Jensenius[35] indicate that the ileum is more important than the jejunum in fat absorption. Others deny any special ability of the ileum for fat absorption,[7, 66] and in fact the work of Gump et al.[26] suggests that the proximal jejunum is especially adapted to neutral fat absorption. Anatomically, there is a greater absorbing surface in the jejunum than in the ileum because of a greater concentration of villi and because of the folds in the mucous membrane of the jejunum. On the other hand, the transit time through the ileum is slower and the chyme reaches the ileum in a more advanced state of digestion, two factors favoring the ileum's efficiency for absorption.

The water soluble vitamins, folic acid, riboflavin, pyridoxine, and ascorbic acid, like carbohydrate, are absorbed quickly from any portion of the small intestine. The fat soluble vitamins are absorbed with the same efficiency as the lipids.

THE ABSORPTION DEFICIT

The deficit responsible for the short bowel malabsorption syndrome is not understood in its entirety. It is probably due to a combination of factors including a deficiency of absorbing area, an increase in transit speed of the chyme over the remaining absorbing surface,[16, 31] and possible deficiencies in digestion.[22, 33] Information as to the relative importance of these factors is scanty.

Some studies suggest that the ileocecal area is of great importance in absorption and that the maintenance of this area aids in preventing the malnutrition seen after massive resection. This has been noted in animals[41, 62] and in patients.[9, 13, 36] Kalser et al.[36] studied transit time, wet stool weight, and percent of fat and nitrogen excreted in patients who had varying lengths and parts of the small intestine resected. Of interest was a group with the terminal ileum and colon intact, but with 8 feet of small bowel removed. This group demonstrated more efficient absorption and slower transit times than did patients with comparable lengths of bowel resected without preservation of the terminal ileum and ileocecal valve. It would seem from these observations that a functioning ileocecal valve and terminal ileum slows transit and enhances absorption.

Booth[9] has remarked further on the importance of the transit time in the short bowel syndrome. He has noted in normal subjects the relatively rapid transit time through the jejunum and the sluggish propulsion in the ileum. Table 6–2 shows some of his data comparing transit times in patients with proximal and distal resection. He has postulated that massive proximal resection is better tolerated than distal resection for this reason. The studies

Table 6–2. Extent of Intestinal Resection and Intestinal Transit Time in Patients with Distal (Cases 1 to 9) or Proximal (Cases 10 and 11) Resection*

Case no.	Age	Extent of intestinal resection	Intestinal transit time†
1	36	Right hemicolectomy and resection of terminal 6 ft. of ileum (pathologic specimens measured)	2 hr.
2	30	Resection of terminal 6 ft. of ileum and cecectomy (pathologic specimens measured)	15 min.
3	40	Right hemicolectomy and resection of 10 ft. of ileum (pathologic specimens measured)	2 hr.
4	48	Right hemicolectomy and resection of all mesenteric small bowel except proximal 6 ft. of jejunum (surgical estimate)	30 min.
5	30	Right hemicolectomy and resection of all mesenteric small bowel except proximal 6 ft. of jejunum (surgical estimate)	20 min.
6	25	Right hemicolectomy and resection of all but proximal 4 ft. of jejunum (surgical and radiologic estimate)	30 min.
7	25	Right hemicolectomy and resection of all but proximal 3 to 4 ft. of jejunum (surgical and radiologic estimate)	30 min.
8	1	Resection of approximately two thirds of distal small intestine—30 in. of proximal jejunum remaining (measured at laparotomy)	30 min.
9	80	Resection of ascending colon and all but proximal 8 in. of jejunum (measured at autopsy)	5 min.
10	71	Resection of proximal 8 ft. of jejunum (pathologic specimen measured)	4 hr.
11	1	Resection of all small intestine except for distal 15 in. of ileum; gastroileal anastomosis (surgical and radiologic estimate)	$1\frac{3}{4}$ hr.

* Adapted from Booth, C. C.: Postgrad. M. J. *37:*727 (Dec.) 1961.

† Intestinal transit time is the time after administration of barium when it reaches the colon. Normal limits vary considerably but are usually between 2 and 6 hours.

of Aberdeen et al.[1] in rats suggest that jejunal fat absorption is decreased by ileal resection, a procedure that decreases jejunal transit time.

Frederick and Craig[22] have suggested that a gastric hypersecretion accompanies small bowel insufficiency and that because of this there is a lowered pH in the proximal bowel that interferes with digestion. Of interest in this regard is an observation by Berman et al.[8] who reported a patient with a resection of the entire mesenteric small intestine except 18 inches of upper jejunum which was anastomosed to the cecum and 6 inches of distal ileum which was sidetracked. These authors found in this case that fat absorption was severely limited but that hydrolysis of oral fat was within normal limits.

SPONTANEOUS RECOVERY

In any evaluation of the short bowel syndrome and particularly in evaluation of therapy of this condition, recognition should be given to the spontaneous improvement in absorptive function shown by the remaining small intestine after massive resection.[45] Althausen et al.[3] demonstrated that the initial deficiencies in glucose, galactose, and water absorption were spontaneously restored to normal in time following resection. Methionine and glycine absorption slowly returned almost to normal, as did butter absorption. These authors found that overall adaptation began a few weeks after the resective procedure.

Possibly related to the spontaneous recovery, as indicated by the studies of Loran and Althausen,[44] are an increase in thickness of all coats of the remaining intestine after resection and an increased rate of cell renewal in the mucosa. Flint[20] reported, in 1912, studies in dogs which demonstrated hypertrophy and hyperplasia of the remaining small intestine and hypertrophy of the remaining villi after massive resection. In addition, Kinney et al.[38] observed a decrease in transit time and hypertrophy and dilatation of the remaining duodenum after resection of the mesenteric small intestine. It is unlikely that absorption from the colon and stomach contributes much to this spontaneous recovery.[19]

CLINICAL CHARACTERISTICS

Since the greater part of all compounds useful to the body economy and most of the water and electrolytes are absorbed by the small intestine, the potential spectrum of the deficiency pattern is almost infinite. Patients deficient in length of small intestine have particular difficulty with fat absorption.[10, 33] Frequently 80 to 90 percent of ingested fat appears in the stools, whereas less than 10 percent is considered within the normal range.

Occasionally a deficiency of the fat soluble vitamins is associated with this steatorrhea.[33] The absorption of amino acids is likely to be impaired but not to as great an extent.[13, 66] Carbohydrate absorption is affected least of all by bowel shortness, and only slightly flattened oral glucose tolerance curves have been noted in patients who have had massive resection.[33]

Net insorption of water is generally accomplished in the ileum and right colon. When this function of these portions of the bowel is not available, deficits in total body water are encountered.[36] However, in spite of deficiencies in total body water, expansion of the extracellular space has been described.[33]

Electrolyte deficiency is not uncommon. Patients with a short small intestine lose large quantities of fluid and electrolytes in diarrheal stools. Hypokalemia[42, 43] and hypocalcemia[36] have been reported in clinically significant and dangerously severe proportions.[18] Levels of calcium of 3.5 mg. per 100 ml. have been observed with subsequent death of the patient.[18] Chronic calcium depletion is often reflected as osteoporosis with normal serum levels.[33] In one case of hypopotassemia[42] there was an associated potassium-losing nephritis of unknown etiology. Frank magnesium deficiency has been reported,[9] at times masked by a normal serum magnesium.[38, 53] Hypophosphatemia is not unknown.[38]

Instances of deficiency of the B vitamins have been recorded.[33, 43, 49] Jackson and Linder[33, 34] and Althausen et al.[2, 3] have noted deficiencies in vitamins A and C in patients with 90 percent or more of the small bowel resected. Hypoprothrombinemia has also been reported.[36]

Anemia is frequent following massive resection and is most often due to a mixed deficiency of folic acid, B_{12}, and iron.[36] However, with only distal resection, isolated B_{12} deficiencies due to loss of the B_{12} absorbing mechanism are observed.[9]

The net result of this malabsorption is evident in weight loss, muscle wasting, osteoporosis, weakness, lassitude and, frequently, death.

PREVENTION

There are three common conditions affecting the small intestine that, when requiring extensive resection, lead to the short bowel syndrome. They are: trauma to the bowel and its vascular supply, infarction of the bowel, and extensive involvement of the small intestine by regional enteritis. Of these, regional enteritis is the most common.[36]

With increasing awareness of the problems connected with deficient arterial supply to the small bowel, the use of emergency massive resection for gangrene should decrease in frequency and elective aortomesenteric bypass or superior mesenteric endarterectomy should become more prevalent. For a fuller discussion of the problems of vascular disease of the small intestine, see Chapter Fifteen. Another cause of bowel infarction is strangulation due to internal herniation and incarceration. This serious complication is also avoidable, but there are difficulties with the early diagnosis of strangulation associated with internal hernias (Chapter Three).

Conservatism in the resective treatment of any small bowel condition is mandatory. In the treatment of extensive forms of regional enteritis, resection should be carried out only for obstruction or fistula, the complications of which are of greater risk to the patient than the development of lesser degrees of the short bowel syndrome. In the treatment of small intestinal polyposis or of traumatic lesions of the small bowel or its mesentery, care must be taken to avoid resection of a segment of bowel beyond the critical length. Frequently with polyposis, the complication of intussusception indicates operative intervention. The conservative procedure of reduction of the intussusception and polypectomy is frequently preferable; resection should be reserved for cases of infarction of the bowel. In cases in which hemorrhage is the indication for surgical intervention, every effort should be made to localize the source of such bleeding so a conservative resection may be carried out.

TREATMENT

SUPPORTIVE

Because of the extreme variability of this syndrome the details of treatment would not be similar in each case. As a general rule a diet high in calories, carbohydrate, and protein should be used.[8, 9, 10, 58] The tolerances for fat in the diet vary greatly among patients with a short bowel. Therefore, the fat content of the diet should be as high as tolerated by the patient without causing an overwhelming diarrhea that accentuates caloric and calcium losses. Supplementation of this diet by vitamins in the form of liquid preparations is important. Electrolyte losses can be replaced by oral or parenteral administration. Magnesium deficiency may require parenteral supplements and should be suspected even if the serum levels of this ion are within normal limits.[38, 53] Calcium replacement is often mandatory.[18] It should be remembered that calcium deficiency can be manifest by osteoporosis without a lowering of the serum calcium levels.[33] Anemias, when present, are frequently due to combined folic acid, B_{12}, and iron deficiencies and are treatable accordingly.[36] The possibility of prothrombin deficiency should not be forgotten and, if present, should be treated with oral or parenteral vitamin K.[36]

The addition to the diet of drugs to prolong the transit time has been used with advantage. Thus, codeine,[38] Kaomagna, or paregoric[10] have been used.

The diet should be administered in frequent feedings so that the available absorbing capacity of the remaining gut is in frequent use.[8] In fact, Kinney et al.[38] obtained an unusual survival in a patient who lost his entire jejunum, ileum, and ascending colon by giving him continuous tube feedings.

Of special recent interest are the studies of Frederick[21] on the use of medium chain fatty acids as supplementation. These fatty acids are more efficiently absorbed than are other lipids.[54] Tween 80 as an emulsification agent to improve fat absorption has not proved useful.[12]

SURGICAL

A number of surgical maneuvers have been tried in the treatment of short bowel malabsorption. Prominent among these has been the reversing of a segment of small intestine to slow the intestinal hurry (Table 6–3), first suggested by Nicoldani.[52] Kirstein[39] and Mall[48] reversed in dogs relatively long segments of the small intestine in continuity. Intestinal obstruction was a prominent result. Since that time, Hammer,[27, 28, 29] Singleton,[59, 60] Sako,[56, 57] and Stahlgren[62] have investigated the results of reversing shorter lengths of small intestine in the dog after massive resection. From this work it is suggested that a reversed loop of 1 to 3 inches in length will prolong survival and increase absorption in the test animals following 75 to 80 percent resection of the small intestine.[6, 27, 28, 37, 56, 57, 62] Reverse peristalsis has been observed in these loops with slowing of intestinal transit. Clinical application of this work has been limited and not well studied (Table 6–4). Gibson et al.[24] in 1962 reported a case of massive resection for gangrene in which 21.5 cm. of jejunum remained and in whom a reversed segment 7.5 cm. in length was used. These authors noted a weight loss from 120 pounds preoperatively to 90 pounds one year later, but at that time the patient was passing one solid stool a day and required no supplemental intake. Two cases of 3-inch reversal with 3 feet of small bowel remaining after resection for ileocolitis were reported by Braasch and Sedgwick.[11] One patient cannot be evaluated, and the other has shown marked improvement one and one quarter years postoperatively. Other reversals of 5 to 8 or 10 inches have been reported for malnutrition,[47, 63] malfunction of ileostomy,[25] or idiopathic diarrhea.[47] All these patients are said to be improved. Two points in the performance of loop reversal bear comment. The first concerns the extreme care that must be taken to avoid twisting and occlusion of the vascular supply to the reversed segment. Second, at least a two-vessel loop must be used to avoid the obstructive features of a Torbey loop.[64] Certainly the reversal technique deserves further careful clinical trial and controlled studies to determine its usefulness.

Other surgical maneuvers have undergone trial in the laboratory. These include the construction of a mechanical impediment to flow by pleating the bowel wall, by tapering the lumen, or by placing constricting Teflon collars

Table 6–3. Laboratory Animal Studies of Loop Reversal

Author and year	Small intestine resection (percent)	Length reversed (inches)	Mortality (percent)	Results: Obstruction	Results: Delay	Results: Absorption	Results: Other
Mall[48]	0	12	100	Yes			
1896		20	100	Yes			
Hammer[29] 1953	0	Entire duodenum			Yes		Gastrojejunal ulcer
Singleton[60]	0	18	0				
1954	0	24	100				
Hammer[27] 1955	75	1					Maintained nutrition
Hammer[28] 1959	80	1–2	0	0	Yes		Survived; maintained weight over 2 yr.
Singleton[59] 1961	All but 36″	9–10	100			I^{131} fat abs. increased 3–4 mo.; then death	
Sako[56] 1962	75	3	100	0	Yes		Prolongs survival but death from inanition
Stahlgren[62]	80–85	5–6	100	Yes		Fat, nitrogen water increased	Nutrition improved
1962	80–85	2–5		0			
Sako[57] 1964	75	3				Fat, protein excretion less	Survival longer without diarrhea
Baldwin-Price[6] 1965	66–70	1.6–2.4		0		Improved I^{131} trioleic acid absorption	Improved weight

Table 6-4. Published Clinical Cases of Loop Reversal

Author and Year	Length of Small Intestine Remaining	Clinical Diagnosis	Length Reversed (*inches*)	Obstruction	Follow-up Time (*years*)	Results
Gibson et al.[24] 1962	8.6 in.	Gangrene	3	0	1	25% weight loss after resection and reversal; 1 solid stool a day; no supplemental intake
Thomas and Jordan[63] 1965	5 ft.	Regional enteritis	6	Markedly dilated proximal jejunum	3	Weight gain from 85 lb. preoperatively to 128 lb. after resection of diseased bowel and loop reversal
Madding et al.[47] 1965	Normal	Idiopathic diarrhea	6	Possibly one episode	1+	Diarrhea abated; gained 18 lb.
	Not stated	Short bowel syndrome	5		Not stated	"Progress excellent"
Braasch and Sedgwick[11] 1965	3 ft.	Regional enteritis	3	0	$1\frac{1}{4}$	Weight gain from 68 to 90 lb.; able to do light housework
	3 ft.	Regional enteritis	3	0	Cannot evaluate	Narcotic addict; has recurrent disease; weight fluctuates

about the bowel.[61] These methods assume that increases in intraluminal pressure caused by partial obstruction are compatible with increased absorption. This supposition is not borne out in one animal study.[5] Still further maneuvers have included vagotomy to slow transit time,[23, 66] intestinal recirculation to more fully utilize the available absorbing surface,[17, 46, 55] and vagotomy and pyloroplasty to provide a more favorable alkaline milieu for digestive activity.[22] Assessment of the results of these maneuvers is difficult owing to problems in obtaining controlled data, especially in clinical cases.

REFERENCES

1. Aberdeen, V., Shepherd, P. A., and Simmonds, W. J.: Concurrent measurement, in unanesthetized rats, of intestinal transport and fat absorption from the lumen. Quart. J. Exper. Physiol. *45:*265–274 (July) 1960.
2. Althausen, T. L., Uyeyama, K., and Simpson, R. G.: Digestion and absorption after massive resection of small intestine; utilization of food from "natural" versus "synthetic" diet and comparison of intestinal absorption tests with nutritional balance studies in patient with only 45 cm. of small intestine. Gastroenterology *12:*795–807 (May) 1949.
3. Althausen, T. L., Doig, R. K., Uyeyama, K., et al.: Digestion and absorption after massive resection of small intestine: II. Recovery of absorptive function as shown by intestinal absorption tests in two patients and consideration of compensatory mechanisms. Gastroenterology *16:*126–139 (Sept.) 1950.
4. Alvarez, W. C.: An Introduction to Gastro-Enterology. Ed. 4. New York, Paul B. Hoeber, 1948.
5. Anderson, R. E., Schmidtke, W. H., and Diffenbaugh, W. G.: Influence of an increased intraluminal pressure on intestinal absorption. Ann. Surg. *156:*276–286 (Aug.) 1962.
6. Baldwin-Price, H. K., Copp, D., and Singleton, A. O., Jr.: Reversed intestinal segments in the management of anenteric malabsorption syndrome. Ann. Surg. *161:*225–230 (Feb.) 1965.
7. Berman, J. K., Brown, H. M., Foster, R. T., and Grisell, T. L.: Massive resection of intestine. J.A.M.A. *135:*918–919 (Dec. 6) 1947.
8. Berman, L. G., Ulevitch, H., Haft, H. H., and Lemish, S.: Metabolic studies of unusual case of survival following resection of all but 18 inches of small intestine; complicated by combined abdominoperineal resection for carcinoma of rectum performed 9 years previously. Ann. Surg. *132:*64–76 (July) 1950.
9. Booth, C. C.: The metabolic effects of intestinal resection in man. Postgrad. M. J. *37:*725–739 (Dec.) 1961.
10. Bothe, F. A., Magee, W. S., and Driscoll, R. H.: Massive resection of small intestine from 15 centimeters distal to ligament of Treitz to within 6 centimeters of ileocecal valve—with 4 year follow-up. Ann. Surg. *140:*755–758 (Nov.) 1954.
11. Braasch, J. W., and Sedgwick, C. E.: Reversed loops in the short bowel syndrome: Preliminary clinical experience. Lahey Clin. Bull. *14:*27–32, 1965.
12. Christensen, N. A., Musgrove, J. E., and Wollaeger, E. E.: Extensive resection of bowel for occlusion of superior mesenteric artery: report of case with postoperative studies of function of gastro-intestinal tract. Proc. Staff Meet., Mayo Clin. *25:*449–459 (Aug. 2) 1950.
13. Clayton, B. E., and Cotton, D. A.: A study of malabsorption after resection of the entire jejunum and the proximal half of the ileum. Gut *2:*18–22 (Mar.) 1961.
14. Coleman, E. P., and Bennett, D. A.: Massive intestinal resection. Am. J. Surg. *59:*429–438 (Mar.) 1943.
15. Croot, H. J.: Extensive resection of small intestine; short review, with 2 new cases. Brit. M. J. *1:*195–198 (Jan. 26) 1952.
16. Cummins, A. J., and Almy, T. P.: Studies on relationship between motility and absorption in human small intestine. Gastroenterology *23:*179–190 (Feb.) 1953.

17. Davis, H. C., Wolcott, M. W., Golder, H. K., and Blum, A. S.: Intestinal recirculation as an aid to absorption; an experimental study. Arch. Surg. *79:*597–599 (Oct.) 1959.
18. DeMuth, W. E., Jr., and Rottenstein, H. S.: Death associated with hypocalcemia after small bowel short circuiting. New England J. Med. *270:*1239–1240 (June 4) 1964.
19. Doolan, P. D., Kyle, L. H., Hess, W., and Phelps, E.: Gastrocolostomy: clinical observations and experimental studies. Gastroenterology *18:*566–578 (Aug.) 1951.
20. Flint, J. M.: The effect of extensive resections of the small intestine. Bull. Johns Hopkins Hosp. *23:*127–144 (May) 1912.
21. Frederick, P. L.: Personal communication.
22. Frederick, P. L., and Craig, T. V.: The effect of vagotomy and pyloroplasty on weight loss and survival of dogs after massive intestinal resection. Surgery *56:*135–143 (July) 1964.
23. Gerwig, W. H., Jr., and Ghaphery, A.: Experimental attempt to delay alimentary transit after small bowel exclusion. Arch. Surg. *87:*34–41 (July) 1963.
24. Gibson, L. D., Carter, R., and Hinshaw, D. B.: Segmental reversal of small intestine after massive bowel resection. Successful case with follow-up examination. J.A.M.A. *182:*952–954 (Dec. 1) 1962.
25. Gillespie, C. E.: Quoted by Madding, G. F., Kennedy, P. A., and McLaughlin, R. T.: Clinical use of antiperistaltic bowel segments. Ann. Surg. *161:*601–604 (Apr.) 1965.
26. Gump, F., Beals, R., and Barker, H. G.: Effect of small intestinal resection on fat absorption. Ann. Surg. *154:*417–423 (Sept.) 1961.
27. Hammer, J. M., Seay, P. H., Hill, E. J., et al.: Intestinal segments as internal pedicle grafts. Arch. Surg. *71:*625–642 (Oct.) 1955.
28. Hammer, J. M., Seay, P. H., Johnston, R. L., et al.: The effect of antiperistaltic bowel segments on intestinal emptying time. Arch. Surg. *79:*537–541 (Oct.) 1959.
29. Hammer, J. M., Visscher, F., and Hill, E. J.: Experimental gastrojejunal ulcers produced by reversing duodenum. Arch. Surg. *67:*23–28 (July) 1953.
30. Haymond, H. E.: Massive resection of the small intestine. An analysis of 257 collected cases. Surg. Gynec. & Obst. *61:*693–705 (Nov.) 1935.
31. Higgins, J. A., Code, C. F., and Orvis, A. L.: The influence of motility on the rate of absorption of sodium and water from the small intestine of healthy persons. Gastroenterology *31:*708–716 (Dec.) 1956.
32. Jackson, W. P. U.: Massive resection of the small intestine. *In* Modern Trends in Gastro-Enterology. Edited by F. A. Jones. New York, Paul B. Hoeber, Inc. 1958, p. 243.
33. Jackson, W. P. U., and Linder, G. C.: Influence of malnutrition on the pancreas; report of case following small gut resection. Metabolism *2:*562–567 (Nov.) 1953.
34. Jackson, W. P. U., and Linder, G. C.: The clinical and metabolic effects of massive intestinal resections. Acta med. scandinav. (Suppl.) *306:*96–106, 1955.
35. Jensenius, H. C.: Results of experimental resections of the small intestine on dogs. Copenhagen, Nyt. Nordisk Forlag, Arnold Busck, 1945.
36. Kalser, M. H., Roth, J. L. A., Tumen, H., and Johnson, T. A.: Relation of small bowel resection to nutrition in man. Proc. World Cong. Gastro. Baltimore, Williams & Wilkins Co., 1958, Vol. 1, pp. 458–468.
37. Keller, J. W., Stewart, W. R., Westerheide, R., et al.: Prolonged survival with paired reversed segment after massive intestinal resection. Arch. Surg. *91:*174–179 (July) 1965.
38. Kinney, J. M., Goldwyn, R. M., Barr, J. S., Jr., and Moore, F. D.: Loss of the entire jejunum and ileum, and the ascending colon. Management of a patient. J.A.M.A. *179:*529–532 (Feb. 17) 1962.
39. Kirstein, A.: Experimentelles zur Pathologie des Ileus. Deutsche med. Wchnschr. *15:*1000–1002 (Dec. 5) 1889.
40. Koeberle, E.: Resection de deux metres d'intestin grele suivie de guerison. Gaz. hebd. de med. *18:*55–58 (Jan. 28) 1881.
41. Kremen, A. J., Linner, J. H., and Nelson, C. H.: Experimental evaluation of nutritional importance of proximal and distal small intestine. Ann. Surg. *140:*439–448 (Sept.) 1954.
42. Levin, H., Zamcheck, N., and Gottlieb, L. S.: Six-year survival following massive intestinal resection with eventual potassium depletion nephropathy. Gastroenterology *40:*818–822 (June) 1961.
43. Linder, A. M., Jackson, W. P. U., and Linder, G. C.: Small gut insufficiency following intestinal surgery; further clinical and autopsy studies of man surviving $3\frac{1}{2}$ years with 7 inches of small intestine. South African J. Clin. Sc. *4:*1–22 (Mar.) 1953.

44. Loran, M. R., and Althausen, T. L.: Cellular proliferation of intestinal epithelia in the rat two months after partial resection of the ileum. J. Biophys. Biochem. Cytol. *7*:667–671 (July) 1960.
45. Lundquist, V. J.: Massive small bowel resection. Minnesota Med. *42*:1059–1064 (Aug.) 1959.
46. Mackby, M. J., Richards, V., Gilfillan, R. S., et al.: Methods of increasing the efficiency of residual small bowel segments; a preliminary study. Am. J. Surg. *109*:32–38 (Jan.) 1965.
47. Madding, G. F., Kennedy, P. A., and McLaughlin, R. T.: Clinical use of anti-peristaltic bowel segments. Ann. Surg. *161*:601–604 (Apr.) 1965.
48. Mall, F.: Reversal of the intestine. Johns Hopkins Hosp. Rep. *1*:93–110, 1896.
49. Marien, B. N., and McCorriston, J. R.: Effects of resection of massive segments of large and small bowel upon fluid and electrolyte balance: an experimental and clinical study. S. Forum (1952) pp. 123–129, 1953.
50. Martin, J. R., Pattee, C. J., Gardner, C., and Marien, B.: Massive resection of small intestine. Canad. M. A. J. *69*:429–433 (Oct.) 1953.
51. Meyer, H. W.: Sixteen-year survival following extensive resection of small and large intestine for thrombosis of the superior mesenteric artery. Surgery *51*:755–759 (June) 1962.
52. Nicoldani, C.: Idee einer Enteroplastik. Wien. med. Presse, *20*:1705–1707 (Dec. 11) 1887.
53. Opie, L. H., Hunt, B. G., and Finlay, J. M.: Massive small bowel resection with malabsorption and negative magnesium balance. Gastroenterology *47*:415–420 (Oct.) 1964.
54. Playoust, M. R., and Isselbacher, K. J.: Studies on the intestinal absorption and intramucosal lipolysis of a medium chain triglyceride. J. Clin. Invest. *43*:878–885 (May) 1964.
55. Redmond, D. C., 2nd, Muraki, T., and Singleton, A. O., Jr.: Effects of recirculating jejunal loops on absorption and transit after massive bowel resection in dogs. S. Forum *15*:291–292, 1964.
56. Sako, K., and Blackman, G. E.: The use of a reversed jejunal segment after massive resection of the small bowel. An experimental study. Am. J. Surg. *103*:202–205 (Feb.) 1962.
57. Sako, K., Gerszi, K., and Marchetta, F. C.: Nutritional effects of a short reversed jejunal segment. Arch. Surg. *89*:1102–1105 (Dec.) 1964.
58. Schwartz, M. K., Medwid, A., Roberts, K. E., et al.: Fat and nitrogen metabolism in patients with massive small bowel resections. S. Forum *6*:385–390, 1955.
59. Singleton, A. O., Jr., Kurrus, F. D., and Donegan, D. W.: The increasing of absorption following massive resections of bowel by means of antiperistaltic bowel segments as measured by radioiodine fat absorption studies. Ann. Surg. *154* (Suppl.):130–132 (Dec.) 1961.
60. Singleton, A. O., Jr., and Rowe, E. B.: Peristalsis in reversed loops of bowel. Ann. Surg. *139*:853–857 (June) 1954.
61. Stahlgren, L. H., Roy, R. H., and Umana, G.: A mechanical impediment to intestinal flow; physiological effects on intestinal absorption. J.A.M.A. *187*:41–44 (Jan. 4) 1964.
62. Stahlgren, L. H., Umana, G., Roy, R., and Donnelly, J.: A study of intestinal absorption in dogs following massive small intestinal resection and insertion of an antiperistaltic segment. Ann. Surg. *156*:483–492 (Sept.) 1962.
63. Thomas, J. F., and Jordan, G. L., Jr.: Massive resection of small bowel and total colectomy: use of reversed segment. Arch. Surg. *90*:781–786 (May) 1965.
64. Torbey, K., and Waddell, W. R.: Function of the colon after removal of anal sphincters and replacement by denervated ileal segments. An experimental study. Ann. Surg. *154*:424–431 (Sept.) 1961.
65. Treves, F.: Lectures on the anatomy of the intestinal canal and peritoneum in man. Brit. M. J. *1*:415–419 (Feb. 28) 1885.
66. Weckesser, E. C., Ankeney, J. L., Portmann, A. F., et al.: Extensive resection of small intestine followed by vagotomy; experimental study of fat and nitrogen excretion on dogs. Surgery *30*:465–476 (Sept.) 1951.
67. Weckesser, E. C., Chinn, A. B., Scott, M. W., Jr., and Price, J. W.: Extensive resection of the small intestine. Am. J. Surg. *78*:706–714 (Nov.) 1949.
68. West, E. S., Montague, J. R., and Judy, F. R.: Digestion and absorption in a man with three feet of small intestine. Am. J. Digest. Dis. *5*:690–692 (Dec.) 1938.
69. Wilkie, W.: Massive resection of small gut—report of case. South African M. J. *24*:516–520 (July 1) 1950.

Chapter Seven

ELECTIVE SHORT-CIRCUITING FOR OBESITY AND HYPERCHOLESTEROLEMIA

OBESITY

The unique position the small intestine plays in the absorption of carbohydrate, protein, and lipids has attracted interest in altering these processes for the treatment of obesity and hyperlipemia.[6] One such surgical alteration is shown in Figure 7–1 in which all of the small intestine except 30 inches of proximal jejunum has been removed from intestinal continuity. In the subject with an artificially produced short bowel there is a decrease in the available absorbing surface and an increase in the transit time past this absorbing surface. These two factors combine to produce fat and protein malabsorption. That this malabsorption can cause elective weight loss in overly obese patients has been demonstrated by several surgeons.[3, 4, 5, 6, 7, 8] A survey of published clinical cases is presented in Table 7–1. It is apparent from these reports that the presence in the fecal stream of only 15 to 30 inches of small intestine allows a progressive loss of weight which tends to level off after the first few months of rapid decline.[6]

Unfortunately, coincident abnormalities of potassium, calcium, magnesium, and sodium metabolism are at times encountered which, if not treated vigorously, can lead to death.[3, 7] Of Lewis'[6] (1966) 10 determinate cases, severe deficiencies of calcium and either magnesium or sodium or both were noted in two. Five others had minimal derangements. Because the area of vitamin B_{12} absorption is bypassed after jejunocolostomy, parenteral supplements of this vitamin must be administered monthly in addition to weekly magnesium sulfate.[6]

Table 7–1. Clinical Experience With Intestinal Shunts in Treatment of Obesity

Author and year	Amount small bowel in continuity	Weight changes (*lb.*)	Follow-up time	Abnormalities or changes noted
Kremen et al.[4] 1954	36″ jejunum to 18″ ileum	Slowly losing weight	"brief"	Weight loss
Lewis et al.[5] 1962	20″ jejunum to transverse colon	237 to 145	2 yr.	Weight loss; serum cholesterol and beta-lipoprotein concentration in blood 50% of normal
	20″ jejunum to cecum	227 to 135	3 yr.	Same as above
Wood and Chremos[9] 1963	18″ jejunum to 8″ ileum	307 to 282 to 311	2½ yr.	Disabling steatorrhea
Payne et al.[7] 1963	15″–20″ jejunum to transverse colon (10 cases)	Lost average 2.4 lb./wk. or 123 lb. loss at 1 yr.		Weight loss; disabling steatorrhea on normal and high fat diets; high blood pressure to normal; elevated blood cholesterol to normal; serum potassium and calcium fell; 5 patients showed clinical hypokalemia; 4 patients showed clinical hypocalcemia; 2 cases had intestinal continuity restored before ideal weight attained
DeMuth and Rottenstein[3] 1964	10″ jejunum to 5″ ileum	300 to 231	7 mo.	Died with tetany; calcium 3.5 mg. per 100 ml.; weight loss
Lewis et al.[6] 1966	20″ to 30″ jejunum to transverse colon (11 cases)	87 to 200 lb. loss	7 to 21 mo.	One case died 5 days postoperatively, unknown cause; one case died 8 mo. postoperatively of embolus; two cases severe, 5 minimal electrolyte abnormalities

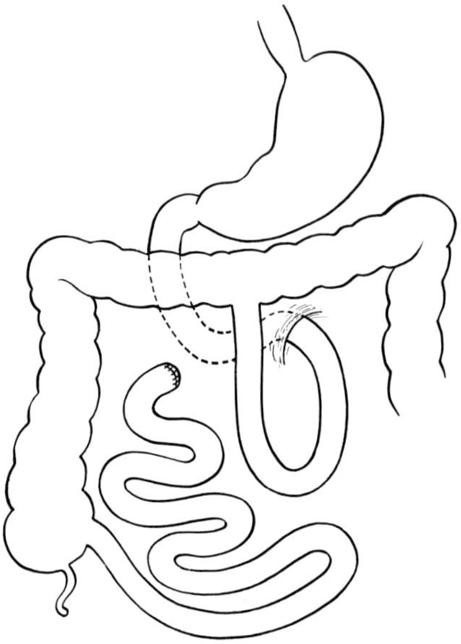

Figure 7–1. Jejunotransverse colostomy for the control of obesity and hyperlipemia.

Other disquieting features of the short-circuiting operation have been reported by Wood and Chremos[9] whose patient increased her diet to maintain her preoperative weight in spite of a disabling steatorrheic diarrhea. Lewis et al.[6] reported frequent nausea and vomiting for varying periods after the shunt was established, and two of their cases have requested reestablishment of intestinal continuity because of weakness.

Of interest is the report of Payne et al.,[7] who reconnected the bypassed small intestine entirely in six cases (Table 7–2) and partially in three (Table 7–3). Of the first group there were four with adequate follow-up. Of these, two promptly returned to their preshunt weights, one had partially returned, and the fourth maintained her ideal weight after three years with a restored intestinal tract. In the second group of three patients who

Table 7–2. Body Weights Before and After Jejunocolic Shunting and After Restoration of *Normal* Intestinal Tract*

ORIGINAL WEIGHT (*lb.*)	WEIGHT AT RESTORATION (*lb.*)	FINAL FOLLOW-UP TIME AFTER RESTORATION (*years*)	WEIGHT AT FINAL FOLLOW-UP (*lb.*)
292	120	?	268
318	193	1/6	201
247	144	1	246
242	124	3	134
391	207	3	280
247	134	3	255

* Adapted from Payne, J. H., et al.: Am. J. Surg. *106*:275 (Aug.) 1963.

Table 7-3. Body Weights Before and After Jejunocolic Shunting and After *Partial* Restoration of Intestinal Tract*

ORIGINAL WEIGHT (*lb.*)	WEIGHT AT PARTIAL RESTORATION (*lb.*)	BOWEL IN CONTINUITY AFTER PARTIAL RESTORATION	FOLLOW-UP TIME AFTER PARTIAL RESTORATION (*years*)	WEIGHT AT FINAL FOLLOW-UP (*lb.*)
256	130	15″ jejunum 42″ ileum	2½	255
243	118	15″ jejunum 20″ ileum	4	160
268	118	15″ jejunum 10″ ileum	⅙	123

* Adapted from Payne, J. H., et al.: Am. J. Surg. *106:*275 (Aug.) 1963.

had their intestinal tract partially restored, one noted return to preshunt weight, one partially returned (32 percent regain of weight lost), and another was not followed for a sufficient period of time.

HYPERCHOLESTEROLEMIA

The bypass procedure has also been suggested and carried out by Buchwald[1] for hypercholesterolemia, since cholesterol is absorbed exclusively in the small intestine and preferentially in the distal half.[2] Buchwald[1] studied rabbits, swine, and humans who had ileal exclusion and found lowered cholesterol absorption and lowered circulating cholesterol levels in test subjects. He also reported four patients who had hypercholesterolemia and atherosclerotic vascular disease on whom ileal exclusion was electively performed. Follow-up observations on these human subjects have not been reported as yet, but it is clear that cholesterol blood levels can be markedly lowered by the bypass procedure.[6, 7] Lewis et al.[6] report the beta-lipoprotein level in blood to be decreased by this procedure but the alpha-lipoprotein levels to remain at the preoperative values.

In summary of this experience it might be said that weight loss of appreciable proportions usually follows intestinal short-circuiting. Concurrently, hypertension and hypercholesterolemia are alleviated, but not without a definite "price" of potentially dangerous abnormalities of calcium, magnesium, sodium, and potassium metabolism[3, 7] and liver dysfunction.[7] After restoration of intestinal continuity, return to preshunt weight usually follows. Nevertheless, when all measures of weight relief fail and when obesity endangers life, a jejunocolic shunt can be effective in the treatment of obesity. It remains to be seen whether the reduction in serum lipids produced by this shunt will have clinical value.

REFERENCES

1. Buchwald, H.: Lowering of cholesterol absorption and blood levels by ileal exclusion. Experimental basis and preliminary clinical report. Circulation *29:*713–720 (May) 1964.
2. Byers, S. O., Friedman, M., and Gunning, B.: Observations concerning production and excretion of cholesterol in mammals; intestinal site of absorption and excretion of cholesterol. Am. J. Physiol. *175:*375–379 (Dec.) 1953.
3. DeMuth, W. E., Jr., and Rottenstein, H. S.: Death associated with hypocalcemia after small bowel short circuiting. New England J. Med. *270:*1239–1240 (June 4) 1964.
4. Kremen, A. J., Linner, J. H., and Nelson, C. H.: Experimental evaluation of nutritional importance of proximal and distal small intestine. Ann. Surg. *140:*439–448 (Sept.) 1954.
5. Lewis, L. A., Turnbull, R. B., Jr., and Page, I. H.: "Short-circuiting" of the small intestine: Effect on concentration of serum cholesterol and lipoproteins. J.A.M.A. *182:*77–79 (Oct. 6) 1962.
6. Lewis, L. A., Turnbull, R. B., Jr., and Page, I. H.: Effects of jejunocolic shunt on obesity, serum lipoproteins, lipids and electrolytes. Arch. Int. Med. *117:*4–16 (Jan.) 1966.
7. Payne, J. H., DeWind, L. T., and Commons, R. R.: Metabolic observations in patients with jejunocolic shunts. Am. J. Surg. *106:*273–289 (Aug.) 1963.
8. Sandblom, P.: Discussion of Kremen et al. (Ref. 4).
9. Wood, L. C., and Chremos, A. N.: Treating obesity by "short-circuiting" the small intestine. J.A.M.A. *186:*63 (Oct. 5) 1963.

Chapter Eight

DIVERTICULAR DISEASE

Diverticular disease of the small intestine is best considered in three clinically oriented groups. These are jejunal diverticulosis, duodenal diverticulum, and Meckel's diverticulum.

For purposes of orientation, duodenal, jejunal, and ileal diverticula are considered false diverticula since they are herniations of the mucosa through the submucosa and muscularis. These are acquired diverticula and are found on the mesenteric side of the bowel wall. Meckel's diverticulum, on the other hand, occurs on the antimesenteric side of the ileum and is a true diverticulum since the walls contain all layers of the small intestine.

False diverticula of the small intestine are most commonly found in the jejunum (Figs. 8–1 and 8–2), but they can occur in the duodenum or

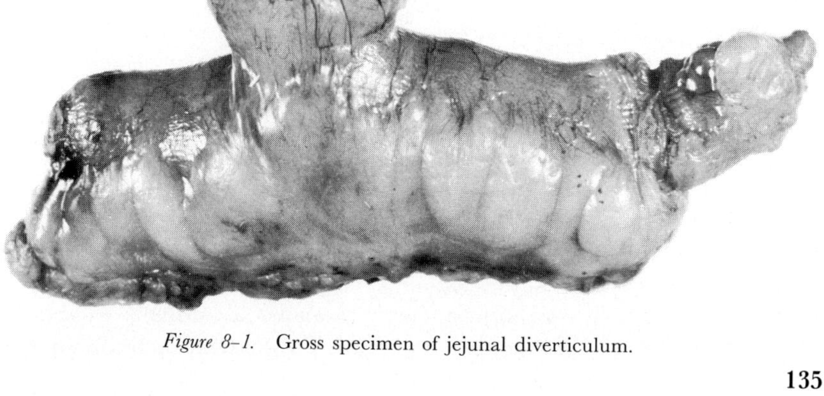

Figure 8–1. Gross specimen of jejunal diverticulum.

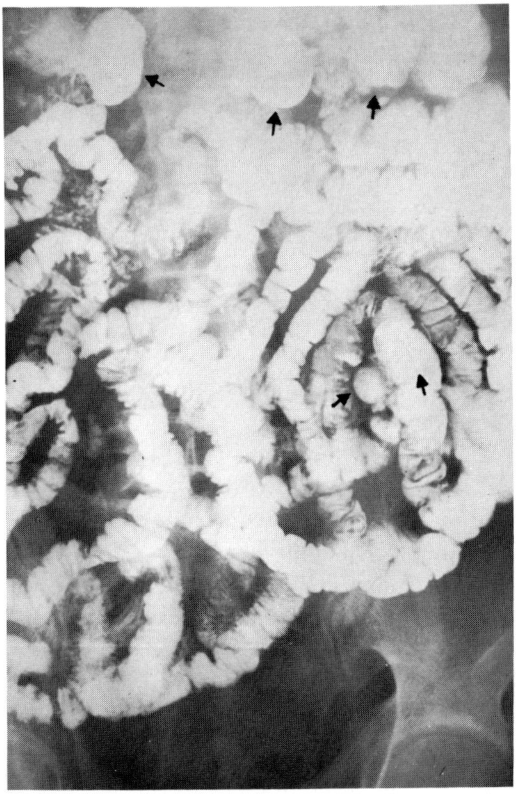

Figure 8–2. Small bowel barium roentgenogram showing jejunal diverticulosis in a patient with malabsorption.

ileum, singly or in combination with others in all three locations.[6, 12] It is not uncommon to have either solitary or more than one diverticulum involving only the duodenum, but it is rare to have a single diverticulum, excepting Meckel's diverticulum, involving just the ileum.[47]

JEJUNAL DIVERTICULOSIS

GENERAL CONSIDERATIONS

The first anatomic description of diverticula of the jejunum was recorded from postmortem material by Cooper[13] in 1807. The clinical features of diverticulosis of the jejunum were first reported by Osler[35] in 1881 when he described the case of a 65-year-old man with 53 jejunal diverticula ranging in size from a cherry to an apple and who complained of colicky abdominal pain and borborygmi. This patient died of "an acute enteric attack" with melena. The first radiological demonstration of jejunal diverticula was reported by Case[9] in 1920.

The diagnosis of jejunal diverticulosis is made usually in patients over the age of 50.[4, 12] There is no sex preponderance.[4, 12] The autopsy incidence of massive diverticulosis of the jejunum varies between 0.1 and 1.0 percent,[4, 36] depending on the technique used for examination. Jejunal diverticulosis is found in 0.06 to 1.0 percent of radiographic examinations.[4]

Theories as to the development of jejunal diverticulosis include many factors such as irregular peristalsis in the segment of bowel involved, spot deficiencies of the longitudinal muscle of the bowel coat, and arteriosclerosis of the mesenteric vessels. None of these mechanisms are particularly acceptable on critical examination. We are inclined to a mechanistic approach to the etiology of jejunal diverticulosis because diverticula are constantly found on the mesenteric side of the bowel near the entrance of the mesenteric vessels.

CLINICAL SYNDROMES AND TREATMENT

A variety of clinical syndromes are associated with jejunal diverticulosis (Table 8–1). Perhaps the most common is that referred to by Altemeier et al.[2] as jejunal dyskinesia which is made up of a number of nonspecific abdominal complaints easily confused with functional bowel disturbances. These include intermittent periumbilical or epigastric pain that lasts for a few hours to a few days. At times the pain is made worse by a change in posture and occasionally is associated with profuse watery stools or nausea and vomiting. Weight loss may be a prominent feature in this chronic bowel syndrome and amounted to more than 7 pounds in 24 of 30 cases reported by Cooke et al.[12]

A striking finding associated with this syndrome has been hypertrophy and dilatation of the bowel wall involved with diverticula.[2] Additionally, there is abnormal hypermotility of the segments of jejunum in the region

Table 8–1. Clinical Syndromes Associated With Jejunal Diverticulosis

Jejunal dyskinesia
Abdominal pain
Bloating
Diarrhea
Nausea
Weight loss
Malabsorption
Steatorrhea
Anemia
Hypoproteinemia
Diverticulitis
Hemorrhage
Intestinal obstruction

of multiple diverticula and immediately distal to the area of diverticulosis. These areas exhibit poor propulsion.

Phillips,[36] in 1953, recognized chronic intestinal obstruction as a manifestation of jejunal diverticulosis and presented several cases with vague symptoms, as just described. He reported several cases that showed dilated and thickened bowel at operation without organic obstruction. Following resection these patients noted marked relief of symptoms with weight gain.

In the treatment of patients with jejunal diverticulosis and vague abdominal symptoms, it should be emphasized that the diverticula are almost always incidental findings.[27] The decision to resect the jejunum under these circumstances may be difficult to make.

A most interesting complication of jejunal diverticulosis is that of malabsorption with steatorrhea and anemia, most commonly of the megaloblastic variety. Megaloblastic anemia associated with certain conditions of the small bowel, chiefly chronic obstruction, was first pointed out by Faber in 1895.[16] Badenoch and Bedford[3] were the first to call attention to malabsorption in association with diverticulosis of the small intestine when they described, in 1954, two patients with three major signs—diverticulosis of the small intestine, megaloblastic anemia, and steatorrhea. One year later, Badenoch et al.[4] (1955) added three further cases and noted that the use of antibiotics improved the deficient absorption of radioactive vitamin B_{12}. These authors believed that this observation gave support to their contention that there was a causal relationship between the diverticula and the deficiency of vitamin B_{12}. Thus, two of their cases were given Aureomycin for one week with decrease in the fecal excretion of radioactive cobalt-tagged B_{12} from 90 to 50 percent of the oral dose.

By 1958 Scudamore et al.[41] were able to document 19 cases of this syndrome in the literature and reported 3 cases of their own. They suggested that the anemia was not true pernicious anemia since 10 of 16 patients tested had free hydrochloric acid on gastric aspiration. They further surmised that this syndrome was not nontropical sprue since the steatorrhea was usually mild, the onset of the diarrhea was sudden, it occurred in elderly patients, there was no deficiency pattern on the small intestinal radiograph, the oral glucose tolerance test was usually normal, and other absorptive defects, if present, were mild. Two of their patients had impaired vitamin B_{12} absorption that was not helped by the addition of intrinsic factor to the therapeutic regimen, but the use of Terramycin was beneficial in this regard. Another confirmatory case of a patient with a 27-pound weight loss and up to 12 bowel movements a day has been reported.[20] In this case there was some elevation of the fat excretion and minimal depression of the vitamin B_{12} absorption. These features and the general clinical condition of the patient were improved greatly by the administration of tetracycline.

A most complete review of the situation with regard to jejunal diverticulosis and malabsorption has been recorded by Cooke et al.[12] They noted the variable and intermittent course of abdominal pain, weight loss, abnormal absorptive patterns, anemia, and neurologic symptoms. Symptomatic anemia was present in only 3 of 30 cases, 1 of which was due to iron deficiency subsequent to a previous gastric resection. However, on laboratory examination 12 had hemoglobin levels of less than 12.8 gm. per 100 ml., and in 4 it was less than 10 gm. per 100 ml. Five had megaloblastic anemia, 3 had been treated with vitamin B_{12}, and 10 had proved or probable megaloblastic anemia at some time in the past. Gastric acidity determinations showed that seven patients, none of whom were anemic, had a histamine-fast achlorhydria. Fourteen patients had evidence of vitamin B_{12} depletion in that the serum vitamin B_{12} levels were low. Nine patients had extremely low radioactive vitamin B_{12} uptakes. Of these, six responded to antibiotic (tetracycline, Aureomycin, or erythromycin) treatment with or without intrinsic factor.

Other evidence of malabsorption included a serum folic acid level below normal in 2 of 16 patients tested, a serum albumin level below 4 gm. per 100 ml. in 20 of 29 patients, a low result in the D-xylose excretion test in 6 of 9 patients, serum calcium levels below 9.4 mg. per 100 ml. in 7 patients, 2 of whom showed evidence of osteomalacia, and fecal fat excretion greater than 6 gm. per day in 9 of 27 tested. Of the 30 patients, neurologic symptoms were present in 12 and were represented by progressive paraplegia, peripheral neuritis with foot drop and ataxia, or subacute combined degeneration of the cord. Of 5 patients with peripheral neuropathy and posterior column disease, 3 were transiently improved by vitamin B_{12} therapy, and 2 improved with antibiotic treatment.

The exact cause of malabsorption in diverticulosis is not known. There is some suggestion that the accumulation of abnormal numbers of bacteria in the diverticula might interfere with absorption, possibly because the organisms have an affinity for vitamin B_{12}.[12] This problem will be further discussed in the consideration of the blind loop syndrome (Chapter Nine).

The treatment of malabsorption related to diverticulosis is oral or parenteral replacement using vitamin B_{12}, folic acid, oral iron, and calciferol, as indicated. The use of antibiotics at times improves vitamin B_{12}, folic acid, and D-xylose absorption. Several cases have been reported which were treated surgically by resection of the involved loops of jejunum.[12] According to Cooke,[12] resection in 5 cases was followed in 4 by improvement in malabsorption to test, but in 1 case there was no change in the steatorrhea or other measures of absorption.

Another complication of jejunal diverticulosis is acute diverticulitis, which can progress to perforation, peritonitis, abscess formation, adhesion formation, or acute intestinal obstruction.[2, 12, 41] Occasionally perforation may occur from traumatic rupture of a diverticulum.[7] Massive bleeding from a jejunal diverticulum has also been reported, although it is rare.[2, 12, 14] Acute or chronic intestinal obstruction may occur as a result of volvulus about the diverticulum,[47] adhesions formed by an old inflammation,[47] or because of enterolith formation within the diverticular sac with subsequent erosion of the enterolith from the sac into the lumen of the small intestine.[47] Other rare complications of diverticular disease include cyst formation caused by occlusion of the mouth of the diverticulum,[21] intussusception with the diverticulum being the leading point,[38] chronic pneumoperitoneum without perforation,[2] the development of carcinoma in the diverticulum,[6, 12] or the entrapment of a foreign body in the diverticulum with obstruction.[2]

The treatment of the mechanical complications of diverticula, such as hemorrhage, perforation, or obstruction, is surgical with resection or bypass of the offending segment of jejunum.

SUMMARY

False, acquired diverticulosis of the small intestine is most frequently seen in the jejunum, but may also be present in the duodenum and, more rarely, in the ileum. It occurs in patients of the older age group, with no sex preponderance. An unknown proportion of patients exhibiting diverticulosis have symptoms ascribable to these diverticula. The symptoms may take the form of chronic intestinal obstruction, with or without mechanical causes, such as volvulus, intussusception, or diverticulitis. Complications may include hemorrhage, traumatic rupture, enterolith formation, and foreign body obstruction. Malabsorption of vitamin B_{12}, fat, protein, folic acid, and other compounds is frequently seen associated with diverticulosis of the jejunum.

The treatment of these complications is resection of the involved diverticulum or segment of intestine or a bypassing procedure to relieve organic obstruction. In cases of malabsorption, parenteral or oral supplementation or antibiotic therapy or both should be utilized.

DUODENAL DIVERTICULUM

GENERAL CONSIDERATIONS

Duodenal diverticula may be classified in three groups: true congenital (rare), primary acquired, and secondary pseudodiverticula, usually due to peptic ulcer (Table 8–2). In addition to these varieties of diverticula, a rare intraluminal duodenal diverticulum has been reported.[17] In the following paragraphs we should like to discuss primary acquired diverticula.

Chomel,[11] in 1710, is credited with first describing a duodenal diverticulum. His particular case occurred in an 80-year-old woman who died of a cerebrovascular accident. This diverticulum contained 22 biliary calculi, and Chomel was mainly interested in the presence of calculi in this unusual location. Bauer,[5] in 1912, reported the first patient to undergo surgical treat-

Table 8–2. Classification of Duodenal Diverticula

I. True congenital diverticula	
	Rare, present from birth
II. Primary diverticula (acquired)	
	No muscle coat; most common usually in second or third portion of duodenum
III. Secondary diverticula (pseudodiverticula)	
	First portion of duodenum due to peptic ulceration or cholecystitis with traction on duodenum

ment of a complicated diverticulum. The patient suffered from chronic nausea and vomiting, and a gastrojejunostomy was performed to sidetrack an obstruction of the duodenum. The patient died in the postoperative period, and at autopsy a diverticulum of the duodenum was found clearly obstructing the duodenum. Case[8, 9] made the first diagnosis of duodenal diverticula before operation or before death; he presented four cases at the scientific exhibit of the American Medical Association in 1913. Forssell and Key[18] reported the first case, in 1916, in which the preoperative diagnosis was made by radiographic methods and the symptomatic diverticulum was successfully removed at surgery.

Primary acquired diverticula[23] almost always occur on the mesenteric side of the duodenum near the entrance of the vascular supply. They are rare in patients under 40 years of age and occur in females slightly more often than in males.[24] The incidence of duodenal diverticula in the general population is between 0.016 and 22 percent,[1] depending on whether the data were obtained from autopsy or x-ray examinations.[24]

Pathologic Anatomy

Duodenal diverticula occur as a single diverticulum in approximately 90 percent of cases. In one large series, 23 percent were associated with jejunal diverticula.[48] They arise most commonly medially near the ampulla of Vater (Fig. 8–3).[24] Tables 8–3 and 8–4 indicate the frequency of their location in relation to the portion of duodenum involved and the position of their orifice in the duodenum.

Occasionally aberrant tissue is found in the diverticulum.[10] Pancreatic acinar tissue and aberrant gastric mucosa associated with peptic ulceration and hemorrhage have been reported.

Clinical Management

Waugh and Johnston[48] have reported 30 cases of surgically treated diverticula of the duodenum, of which only 8 had symptoms directly referable to the diverticulum. During the same time period as this study, the diag-

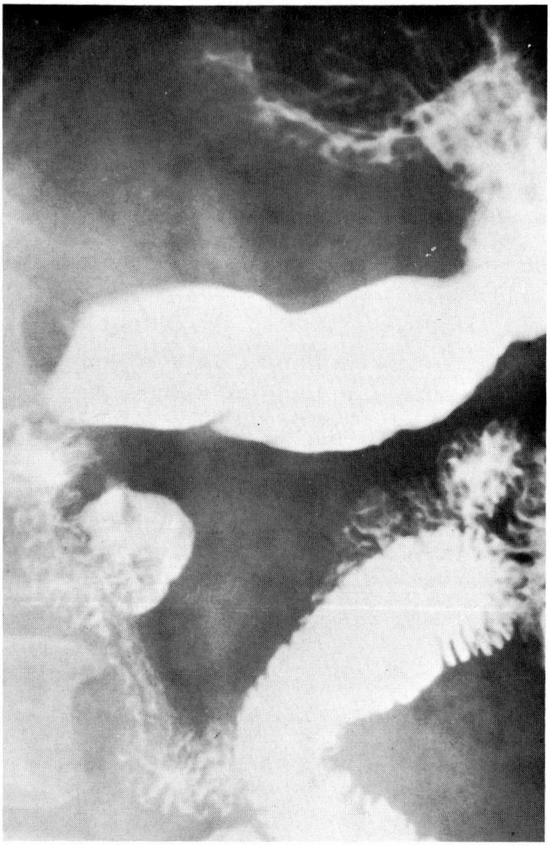

Figure 8–3. Duodenal diverticulum near the ampulla of Vater as shown on upper gastrointestinal study.

Table 8–3. Frequency of Location of Duodenal Diverticula as to Portion of Duodenum*

PORTION OF DUODENUM	PERCENT FREQUENCY
1	6
2	65
3	30
4	8

* Adapted from Jones, T. W., and Merendino, K. A.: Surgery *48:*1076 (Dec.) 1960. Note total frequency greater than 100 percent due to 10 percent incidence of multiple diverticula.

Table 8-4. Position of Orifice on Duodenum in Horizontal Plane*

Position	Percent frequency
Medial	88
Lateral	4
Anterior	22
Posterior	8

* Adapted from Jones, T. W., and Merendino, K. A.: Surgery *48:*1076 (Dec.) 1960. Note total frequency greater than 100 percent due to 10 percent incidence of multiple diverticula.

nosis of duodenal diverticulum was made 525 times by their associates. This series gives an indication of the rarity of symptomatic diverticula. The clinician is often faced with deciding whether the diverticulum is responsible for the disability in a patient with both a duodenal diverticulum and indigestion. It has been emphasized that one must be most cautious in ascribing these functional complaints to the diverticulum.[10, 24, 48] Vague indigestion, weight loss, nausea and vomiting, diarrhea, and tenderness on palpation of the upper abdomen have all been ascribed to duodenal diverticula. However, it seems likely that only the symptoms due to the serious complications of diverticula are of importance (Table 8-5). In deciding which diverticula are symptomatically significant, Mahorner[30] suggested that the larger diverticula which retain barium should be excised. Cattell and Mudge[10] recommended excision in those symptomatic cases in which the diverticulum did not empty in six hours after a barium meal, was tender to palpation, and was of large size. Major complications of diverticula which make laparotomy advisable include the development of neoplasms in the diverticulum (leiomyosarcoma,[32] carcinoma,[43] leiomyoma,[15] and fibroma[46]) hemorrhage,[25] perforation by peroral suction biopsy,[19] duodenocolic fistula,[37] common duct obstruction, and acute pancreatitis.[34]

Operative Treatment

The preferred operative treatment is excision of the diverticulum. Extreme care must be exercised because of the danger of postoperative pancreatitis,

Table 8-5. Complications of Duodenal Diverticula*

Jaundice with obstruction of the bile duct	Perforation
Cholangitis	Ulceration
Acute or chronic pancreatitis	Malignancy
Partial duodenal obstruction	Massive hemorrhage
Diverticulitis and peridiverticulitis	Fistulas into the common bile duct
Duodenocolic fistula	

* Adapted from Jones, T. W., and Merendino, K. A.: Surgery *48:*1079 (Dec.) 1960.

since frequently the diverticulum is closely associated with the pancreas. Other methods of treatment include inversion of the diverticulum or posterior gastrojejunostomy with vagotomy to bypass the duodenum. This latter procedure is particularly useful if severe inflammation obscures the field or if the diverticulum is closely associated with the ampulla of Vater and cannot be resected without damage to the bile or pancreatic ducts.[10] MacLean[29] has emphasized certain technical features in the surgical treatment of diverticula. In those cases in which the diverticulum is embedded in the pancreas, he advises duodenotomy and insertion of the surgeon's finger within the diverticulum as a guide for excision of the diverticulum. Mahorner[30] has emphasized intubation of the common duct as an aid in avoiding injury to this structure during excision of diverticula around the ampulla of Vater. In locating duodenal diverticula at surgery, he also recommended insufflation of the duodenum and the diverticula to aid in their recognition. Another maneuver, as used by Waugh and Johnston[48] in the excision of diverticula, is the obliteration of the neck of the diverticulum from inside the bowel. If diverticulectomy is elected, the surgeon must be careful not to remove all of the neck of the diverticulum, since the tissues of the neck are most useful in obtaining a watertight closure of the duodenal defect.

RESULTS OF SURGICAL TREATMENT

The mortality for resection of duodenal diverticula, as reported in the literature, is between 5 and 10 percent.[24] Postoperative deaths are usually due to injury of the ampulla, to pancreatitis, or to leakage of the duodenum at the point of closure. Because of this, drainage of the abdomen is mandatory and, as mentioned earlier, extreme care in dealing with the bile duct, the pancreas, and the closure of the neck of the diverticulum is essential. Waugh and Johnston[48] reported 20 operated cases, 1 of which was complicated by stricture of the bile duct, another by pancreatitis, 2 by duodenal fistulas, 1 by subhepatic abscess, and 1 case in which the bile duct had to be transplanted when closure of the neck of the duodenal diverticulum compromised the lumen of the duct. These complications led to 2 deaths, 1 from renal failure and another from peritonitis from leakage. In 10 cases, the removal of the diverticulum was the only significant procedure accomplished. One of these patients was lost to follow-up, and 2 died postoperatively. Of 7 remaining patients, 2 had complete relief of digestive symptoms and 3 had poor results. Two patients were operated on for hemorrhage; one was relieved, and in the other a gastric ulcer was overlooked, and subsequently hemorrhage again occurred.

Cattell and Mudge[10] reported 25 operated cases with 2 deaths due to pancreatitis. In 17 cases the only definitive operative procedure was excision of the diverticulum. In 9 the result was excellent, in 3 fair, and in 5 poor.

SUMMARY

Duodenal diverticula are frequent abnormalities of the duodenum. Among those that are symptomatic (rare), most disability is evidenced by indigestion and postcibal pain or by the complications of pressure of the diverticulum on the surrounding structures. Surgical treatment of the duodenal diverticulum is rarely indicated, and the need for this must be thoroughly documented before it is carried out. The preferred surgical treatment is excision, using a variety of maneuvers designed to protect the adjacent structures and to prevent leakage at the suture line.

MECKEL'S DIVERTICULUM

Meckel's diverticula have incited interest among clinicians since Meckel's first description of this anomaly.[31] Within the last decade three extensive reviews of this subject have been published.[42, 45, 49]

Meckel's diverticula are true diverticula and are located usually on the antimesenteric edge of the ileum. In a series reported by Weinstein et al.[49] the distance from the diverticulum to the ileocecal valve varied from 1 inch to 6 feet with an average of 21.5 inches. The diverticula in this series varied

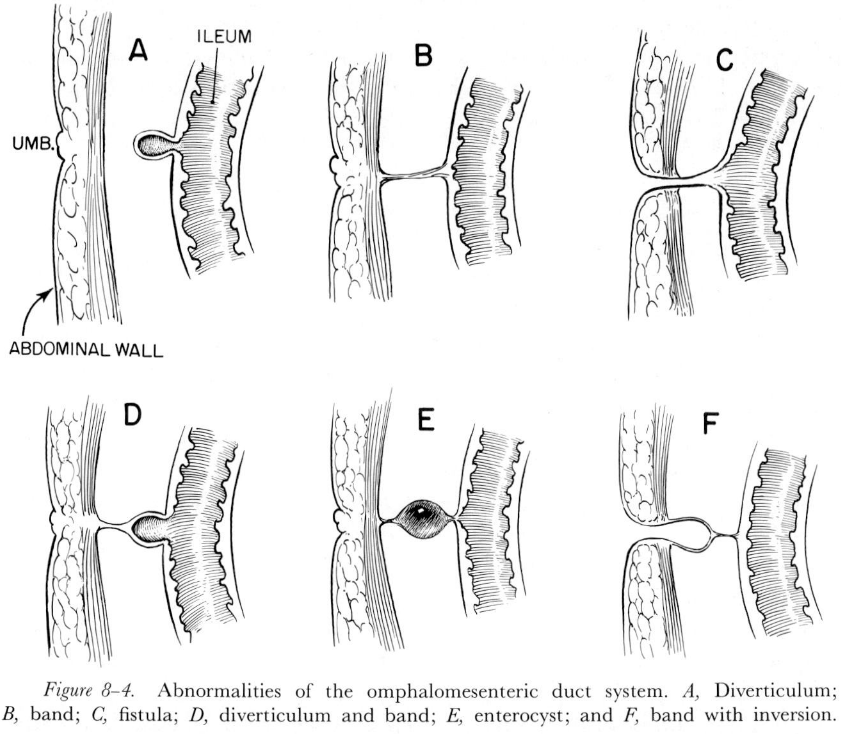

Figure 8–4. Abnormalities of the omphalomesenteric duct system. *A,* Diverticulum; *B,* band; *C,* fistula; *D,* diverticulum and band; *E,* enterocyst; and *F,* band with inversion.

Table 8–6. Anatomic Types of Meckel's Diverticulum*

	PERCENT
Antimesenteric with closed distal end	82.5
Partial obliteration with fibrous cord to umbilicus	10.0
Umbilical fistula	6.0
Giant forms (up to 100 cm. long)	0.5
Umbilical polyp	0.5
Simple intramesenteric	0.5
Cyst formation of cord	Rare

* Adapted from Thompson, J. E.: Ann. Surg. *105*:44–45 (Jan.) 1937.

in size from 1.0 cm. by 0.3 cm. to 11.0 cm. by 3.5 cm. The incidence of this anomaly is variously reported to be between 0.3 and 3.0 percent.[45] Males outnumber females 3 to 1.

Occasionally there is a familial occurrence of Meckel's diverticulum. Four members in one family and three previously reported families with an increased occurrence have been collected by Lewenstein and Levenson.[28]

Embryologically, Meckel's diverticulum is an abnormality of the omphalomesenteric duct system that connects the yolk sac with the intestinal tract at the junction of the foregut and hindgut. This tract is normally completely obliterated by the fifth to seventh week of gestation. Failure of obliteration may result in a diverticulum, fistula, enterocyst, or band as shown in Figure 8–4. Heterotopic tissue occurs in one third of Meckel's diverticula and may be gastric, duodenal, jejunal, pancreatic, acinar, or colonic. Table 8–6 lists the anatomical derangements and the frequency with which they are associated with Meckel's diverticula.

COMPLICATIONS

The complications of Meckel's diverticulum have been outlined by Moses[33] and Veith and Botsford,[45] who compiled 1810 cases (Table 8–7). Hemorrhage is the most common complication. It is most frequently seen in children, and is usually associated with gastric mucosa in the diverticulum. Schaaff[40] analyzed the fluid from a diverticulum containing gastric mucosa and found 40 units of free acid and 70 units of total acid. In Weinstein's series, hemorrhage occurred in 63 patients.[49] Of these, 39 had ulcers; 31 were peptic, and 8 were inflammatory. The usual location for such an ulcer associated with Meckel's diverticulum is at the junction of the ectopic gastric mucosa with the ileal mucosa. Clinically, the bleeding episodes associated with peptic ulceration are characterized by their infrequency, with long intervals between episodes. In resecting the Meckel's diverticulum for this complication, the surgeon must do a sleeve resection of the ileum to be sure that the bleeding point is removed.[45]

Intestinal obstruction resulting from Meckel's diverticulum is usually

Table 8–7. Complications of Meckel's Diverticulum

	PERCENT
Hemorrhage	29.9
Bowel obstruction	23.3
Inflammation	14.2
Perforation	13.2
Littre's hernia	10.4
Umbilical fistula; Foreign body; Umbilical polyp; Malignant tumor; Tuberculosis; Typhoid perforation; Prolapse through navel; Omphalocele; Traumatic perforation	9.0

the result of inflammation of the diverticulum, adhesions from the tip of the diverticulum to adjacent loops of intestine, or twisting of the intestine about a fibrous cord from the diverticulum to the abdominal wall. At times there is intussusception of the diverticulum,[22] frequently from a tumor in the tip which provides the leading point.[42]

In cases of Meckel's diverticulitis, gastric mucosa is found in approximately 38 percent and may be responsible for the development of inflammation.[49] Perforation[44, 45] may be a result of gangrenous diverticulitis, peptic ulcer, or the presence of a foreign body in the diverticulum.[39]

Littre's hernia, or any hernial sac containing a Meckel's diverticulum, is uncommon. It has been found with inguinal, femoral, or umbilical hernias.

Neoplasms originating in Meckel's diverticula (Table 8–8) have been reviewed by Soderlund[42] and by Lechner and Chamblin.[26] By 1962 there were 19 cases of carcinoid tumors in a Meckel's diverticulum recorded in

Table 8–8. Neoplasms of Meckel's Diverticulum

- Benign
    - Lipoma
    - Myoma
    - Fibroma
    - Neurofibroma
    - Angioma
    - Leiomyoma
    - Enterocystoma
    - Adenoma
    - Mesodermal tumor
- Malignant
    - Carcinoid
    - Carcinoma
    - Sarcoma
        - Spindle cell
        - Fibrosarcoma
        - Leiomyosarcoma

the literature.[26] Ten were found at laparotomy and 9 at postmortem examination. Of the 10 found at laparotomy, 4 were associated with symptoms due to metastasis, and 4 were incidental findings. One case in this group had the flushing symptoms of the carcinoid syndrome. Twenty-six percent had metastasis, a figure similar to that for carcinoids of the small intestine in general.

Other complications of Meckel's diverticula are associated with congenital anomalies of the omphalomesenteric duct system and are seen most frequently in children.

If a Meckel's diverticulum is encountered at laparotomy, Veith and Botsford[45] thought it should be excised. We agree with this thesis and perform segmental excision of the ileum with end-to-end anastomosis.

REFERENCES

1. Ackerman, W.: Diverticula and variations of the duodenum. Ann. Surg. *117:*403–413 (Mar.) 1943.
2. Altemeier, W. A., Bryant, L. R., and Wulsin, J. H.: The surgical significance of jejunal diverticulosis. Arch. Surg. *86:*732–745 (May) 1963.
3. Badenoch, J., and Bedford, P. D.: Massive diverticulosis of the upper intestine presenting with steatorrhea and megaloblastic anaemia. Transactions of the Association of Physicians of Great Britain and Ireland. Quart. J. Med. *23:*462, 1954.
4. Badenoch, J., Bedford, P. D., and Evans, J. R.: Massive diverticulosis of small intestine with steatorrhoea and megaloblastic anaemia. Quart. J. Med. *24:*321–330 (Oct.) 1955.
5. Bauer, T.: Über das duodenaldivertikel. Wien. klin. Wchnschr. *25:*879–880 (June) 1912.
6. Benson, R. E., Dixon, C. F., and Waugh, J. M.: Nonmeckelian diverticula of the jejunum and ileum. Ann. Surg. *118:*377–393 (Sept.) 1943.
7. Butler, R. W.: Traumatic rupture of intramesenteric diverticula of the jejunum. Brit. J. Surg. *25:*277–279 (Oct.) 1937.
8. Case, J. T.: Roentgen observations on the duodenum with special reference to lesions beyond the first portion. Am. J. Roentgenol. N.S. *3:*314–326 (June) 1916.
9. Case, J. T.: Diverticula of small intestine, other than Meckel's diverticulum. J.A.M.A. *75:*1463–1470 (Nov. 27) 1920.
10. Cattell, R. B., and Mudge, T. J.: Surgical significance of duodenal diverticula. New England J. Med. *246:*317–324 (Feb. 28) 1952.
11. Chomel, J. B.: Report of a case of duodenal diverticulum containing gallstones. *From* Histoire de l'Academie Royale Des Sciences à Paris. 1710, pp. 48–50.
12. Cooke, W. T., Cox, E. V., Fone, D. J., et al.: The clinical and metabolic significance of jejunal diverticula. Gut *4:*115–131 (June) 1963.
13. Cooper, A.: The anatomy and surgical treatment of crural and umbilical hernia. London, Longman, 1807.
14. Coran, A. G., and Brooks, J. R.: Gastrointestinal bleeding from jejunal diverticulosis. J.A.M.A. *191:*675–676 (Feb. 22) 1965.
15. Dunstan, E., Lowance, M. I., and Jones, E. C.: The clinical importance of duodenal diverticula. South. M. J. *42:*460–467 (June) 1949.
16. Faber, K. I.: Perniciøs anaemia som følge af tarmlidelse. Hospitalstid. *4:*601–615, 1895.
17. Figiel, S. J., and Figiel, L. S.: Intraluminal duodenal diverticulum: report of a case. Am. J. Digest. Dis. *8:*460–462 (May) 1963.
18. Forssell, G., and Key, E.: Ein Divertikel an der pars descendens duodeni mittels Röntgenuntersuchung diagnostiziert und operativ entfernt. Fortschr. Geb. Röntgenstrahlen *24:*48–57, 1916.
19. Gibbs, D. D., and Keynes, W. M.: Perforation of a duodenal diverticulum by peroral suction biopsy. Gastroenterology *44:*685–688 (May) 1963.
20. Goldstein, F., Cozzolino, H. J., and Wirts, C. W.: Diarrhea and steatorrhea due to a

large solitary duodenal diverticulum. Report of a case. Am. J. Digest. Dis. *8:*937–943 (Nov.) 1963.
21. Gordinier, H. C., and Sampson, J. A.: Diverticulitis (not Meckel's) causing intestinal obstruction. Multiple mesenteric (acquired) diverticula of the small intestine. J.A.M.A. *46:*1585–1590 (May 26) 1906.
22. Harmston, G. J., and Cragun, W. E.: Acute intussusception due to torsion of Meckel's diverticulum. Rocky Mountain M. J. *46:*291–293 (Apr.) 1949.
23. Horton, R. E., and Peacock, J. H.: Lateral duodenal diverticula; a report of two cases. Brit. J. Surg. *40:*577–578 (May) 1953.
24. Jones, T. W., and Merendino, K. A.: The perplexing duodenal diverticulum. Surgery *48:*1068–1084 (Dec.) 1960.
25. Langman, M. J. S.: Duodenal diverticula and haemorrhage. Gut *4:*30–31 (Mar.) 1963.
26. Lechner, G. W., and Chamblin, S. A., Jr.: Carcinoid tumors of Meckel's diverticula. Am. J. Surg. *103:*266–268 (Feb.) 1962.
27. Lee, R. E., and Finby, N.: Jejunal and ileal diverticulosis. Arch. Int. Med. *102:*97–102 (July) 1958.
28. Lewenstein, H. J., and Levenson, S. S.: Familial occurrence of Meckel's diverticulum. New England J. Med. *268:*311–312 (Feb. 7) 1963.
29. MacLean, N. J.: Duodenal diverticulitis. Ann. Surg. *85:*73–83 (Jan.) 1927.
30. Mahorner, H.: Diverticula of duodenum; report of 8 surgical cases. Ann. Surg. *133:*697–707 (May) 1951.
31. Meckel, J. F.: Beitrage zur vergleichenden Anatomie. Leipzig, Carl Heinrich Reclam, 1808, p. 91.
32. Mendillo, A. J., and Koufman, W. B.: Diverticulum and sarcoma of the duodenum: report of a case. New England J. Med. *219:*432–433 (Sept. 22) 1938.
33. Moses, W. R.: Meckel's diverticulum; report of 2 unusual cases. New England J. Med. *237:*118–122 (July 24) 1947.
34. Ogilvie, R. F.: Duodenal diverticula and their complications with particular reference to acute pancreatic necrosis. Brit. J. Surg. *28:*362–379 (Jan.) 1941.
35. Osler, W.: Notes on intestinal diverticula. Ann. Anat. Surg. *4:*202–207, 1881.
36. Phillips, J. H. C.: Jejunal diverticulosis; some clinical aspects. Brit. J. Surg. *40:*350–354 (Jan.) 1953.
37. Rhodes, A., and Williams, J. A.: Benign duodenocolic fistula. Surg. Gynec. & Obst. *123:*1071–1074 (Nov.) 1966.
38. River, L. P., and Silverstein, J.: Diverticula of small intestine; report of case of jejunal diverticulum. J. Internat. Coll. Surgeons *15:*347–351 (Mar.) 1951.
39. Roessel, C. W.: Perforation of Meckel's diverticulum by foreign body: case report and review of the literature. Ann. Surg. *156:*972–975 (Dec.) 1962.
40. Schaaff, G.: Beitrag zur bildung des ulcus pepticum im meckelschen divertikel. Deutsche Ztschr. f. Chir. *238:*78–87 (Nov.) 1932.
41. Scudamore, H. H., Hagedorn, A. B., Wollaeger, E. E., et al.: Diverticulosis of the small intestine and macrocytic anemia with report of two cases and studies on absorption of radioactive vitamin B_{12}. Gastroenterology *34:*66–82; discussion, 83–84 (Jan.) 1958.
42. Soderlund, S.: Meckel's diverticulum. A clinical and histologic study. Acta chir. scandinav. *248* (Suppl.):1–233, 1959.
43. Strode, J. E.: Radical duodenopancreatectomy; report of successful resection of carcinoma of duodenal diverticulum involving head of pancreas. Surgery *18:*115–129 (July) 1945.
44. Thompson, J. E.: Perforated peptic ulcer in Meckel's diverticulum. Report of a case occurring intramesenteric. Ann. Surg. *105:*44–55 (Jan.) 1937.
45. Veith, F. J., and Botsford, T. W.: Disease of Meckel's diverticulum in adults. Am. Surgeon *28:*674–677 (Oct.) 1962.
46. Vigna, A.: Quoted by Feldman, M.: The association of duodenal diverticula with pancreatic disease, with special reference to carcinoma of the pancreas. Am. J. Gastroenterology *28:*615–620 (Dec.) 1957.
47. Walker, R. M.: Complications of acquired diverticulosis of jejunum and ileum. Brit. J. Surg. *32:*457–463 (Apr.) 1945.
48. Waugh, J. M., and Johnston, E. V.: Primary diverticula of duodenum. Ann. Surg. *141:*193–200 (Feb.) 1955.
49. Weinstein, E. C., Cain, J. C., and ReMine, W. H.: Meckel's diverticulum: 55 years of clinical and surgical experience. J.A.M.A. *182:*251–253 (Oct. 20) 1962.

Chapter Nine

BLIND LOOP SYNDROME

Surgically constructed blind intestinal loops, intestinal strictures, or partially obstructed intestinal anastomoses are at times associated with malabsorption and, in the case of blind loops, with a variety of other clinical abnormalities. This syndrome is very similar to that seen in cases of jejunal diverticulosis.

HISTORICAL DEVELOPMENT

Faber[12] in 1895 was the first to point out that an anemia consistent with pernicious anemia is sometimes found in patients with intestinal stricture of unknown etiology. The association of this clinical picture with a surgically produced blind loop was first reported by Little et al.[18] in 1929. In 1929 Meulengracht[19] suggested that the anemia seen with an intestinal stricture might be on the basis of a stasis infection in the lumen of the proximal bowel. Holm[17] in 1933 reproduced this malabsorption syndrome in dogs and found in addition that two of the animals developed perforation of the sidetracked loop and that in others at sacrifice there were numerous ulcers scattered throughout the mucosa of this segment of the intestine. In 1939 Barker and Hummel[2] collected the existing cases in the literature and added two of their own to report a total of 51 patients with macrocytic anemia associated with intestinal strictures and anastomoses. They pointed out that treatment of the anemia by liver extract was generally effective, as was corrective surgery. In 1953 Clawson[5] reviewed the literature and concluded that not only could surgically constructed blind loops cause megaloblastic or microcytic anemia, but they could be responsible for crampy abdominal pain, fatigue, nausea, distention or mass, episodic diarrhea, weakness, and an inability to gain weight. He presented a case illustrating dilatation of a blind loop with ulceration and anemia occurring 10 years after a side-to-side anastomosis. In agreement with this viewpoint were Heifetz and Senturia,[15] who recommended resection with end-to-end anastomosis in symptomatic cases.

CLINICAL FEATURES

It is likely that thousands of side-to-side anastomoses have been performed. However, disability due to the blind pouch syndrome is rare, probably because pouches distal to side-to-side anastomoses are not large at the time of their construction and do not usually enlarge later.

Steatorrhea

Clinically significant steatorrhea occurs in approximately one third of cases with the blind loop syndrome[1] and can be reproduced in the laboratory animal.[7] It would seem that the steatorrhea is associated with an inefficient absorption of fat, since hydrolysis of carbon-14 labeled Triolein has been shown to be normal and since orally administered radioactive fats are poorly absorbed.[7] The malabsorption features of the blind loop syndrome also include hypoalbuminemia and inconsistent impairment of xylose absorption.[1, 6, 8]

Anemia

The anemia that occurs with intestinal stagnation is almost always macrocytic. However, if ulceration occurs in the blind pouch, the anemia can be microcytic from blood loss.[16] Cameron et al.[4] have reported 61 cases of intestinal stricture and anemia, of which 33 were associated with glossitis, 12 had subacute combined degeneration of the cord, 19 were icteric, and 60 showed macrocytosis. Of these 61 cases, 24 had free hydrochloric acid in the stomach, 20 had no free hydrochloric acid, and in 17 there was no record of the acidity. Of 25 cases treated surgically by resection, 11 died postoperatively, and in 8 the anemia was cured by the operative procedure. In six patients there was no benefit, but in four of these there was progression of the original disease, and in one the operation was technically unsuccessful.

This syndrome is due to a deficiency of vitamin B_{12} secondary to impaired absorption. The resulting peripheral blood and bone marrow are indistinguishable from those in addisonian pernicious anemia. Thus, the Schilling test shows low urinary excretion of radioactivity, and serum vitamin B_{12} levels are depressed.[14] The administration of liver extract,[4] folic acid, or vitamin B_{12} incites a hematologic response in the therapy of this syndrome.[14]

It is interesting, relative to the etiology of vitamin B_{12} malabsorption, to observe that whereas the oral administration of neomycin did not result in any increase in vitamin B_{12} absorption,[11] the use in patients[9, 14, 21] and in the laboratory animal[9, 20, 22] of an oral broad-spectrum antibiotic did result in alleviation of the megaloblastic anemia. It is also reported that surgical removal of these blind loops or correction of the partial obstruction results in cure of the malabsorption.[9, 14, 21]

Because of the ameliorating effects of antibiotics, it is natural that efforts be directed to implicate the bacteria of the intestine as the causative agent. Donaldson[8] has critically examined this theory. It is true that the contents of partially obstructed blind loops and the bowel proximal to an obstruction contain high titers of viable bacteria.[13] In addition, Donaldson, Corrigan, and Natsios[10] in 1962 demonstrated that bacteria were capable of removing vitamin B_{12} from incubation media. Studies have not been made, however, that correlate the disappearance of these bacteria with improvement of vitamin B_{12} absorption following the administration of broad-spectrum antibiotics.

SURGICAL FEATURES

Knowledge of the potentialities of blind loops and intestinal strictures to produce malabsorption is important to the surgeon. It is probable that only a few side-to-side anastomoses are associated with blind loops and this clinical syndrome, but if side-to-side anastomoses are used, they should be so constructed as to minimize the possibility of blind loop formation.[3] Excisional therapy of strictures or blind loops where they are clinically significant should be carried out.[9, 14, 21]

REFERENCES

1. Badenoch, J.: The blind-loop syndrome. *In* Modern Trends in Gastro-Enterology. Edited by F. A. Jones. New York, Paul B. Hoeber, 1958, pp. 231–242.
2. Barker, W. H., and Hummel, L. E.: Macrocytic anemia in association with intestinal strictures and anastomoses; review of literature and report of 2 new cases. Bull. Johns Hopkins Hosp. *64:*215–256 (Apr.) 1939.
3. Black, B. M., and McEachern, C. G.: Redundant blind segments of intestine following side-to-side anastomosis with division of bowel; report of 5 cases. Surg. Gynec. & Obst. *86:*177–182 (Feb.) 1948.
4. Cameron, D. G., Watson, G. M., and Witts, L. J.: Clinical association of macrocytic anemia with intestinal stricture and anastomosis. Blood *4:*793–802 (July) 1949.

5. Clawson, D. K.: Side-to-side intestinal anastomosis complicated by ulceration, dilatation, and anemia: physiologically unsound procedure; review of literature and presentation of case. Surgery *34:*254–257 (Aug.) 1953.
6. Doig, A., and Girdwood, R. H.: The absorption of folic acid and labelled cyanocobalamin in intestinal malabsorption, with observations on the faecal excretion of fat and nitrogen and the absorption of glucose and xylose. Quart. J. Med. *29:*333–374 (July) 1960.
7. Donaldson, R. M., Jr.: Inhibition of intestinal metabolism of fatty acid in the blind-loop syndrome. Clin. Research *11:*291 (Oct.) 1963.
8. Donaldson, R. M., Jr.: Normal bacterial populations of the intestine and their relation to intestinal function. New England J. Med. *270:*938–945 (Apr. 30); 994–1001 (May 7); 1050–1056 (May 14) 1964.
9. Donaldson, R. M., Jr.: Studies on the pathogenesis of steatorrhea in the "blind loop syndrome." Abstracts of the Annual Meeting of the American Gastroenterological Association. Gastroenterology *46:*738 (June) 1964.
10. Donaldson, R. M., Jr., Corrigan, H., and Natsios, G.: Malabsorption of CO^{60}-labeled cyanocobalamin in rats with intestinal diverticula. II. Studies on contents of the diverticula. Gastroenterology *43:*282–290 (Sept.) 1962.
11. Doscherholmen, A., and Hagen, P. S.: Absorption of CO^{60} labeled vitamin B_{12} in intestinal blind loop megaloblastic anemia. J. Lab. & Clin. Med. *44:*790–791 (Nov.) 1954.
12. Faber, K. I.: Perniciøs anaemia som følge af tarmlidelse. Hospitalstid. *1:*601–615, 1895.
13. Goldstein, F., Wirts, C. W., and Josephs, L.: The bacterial flora of the small intestine. Abstract from Annual Meeting of the American Gastroenterological Association. Gastroenterology *42:*755–756 (June) 1962.
14. Halsted, J. A., Lewis, P. M., and Gasster, M.: Absorption of radioactive vitamin B_{12} in syndrome of megaloblastic anemia associated with intestinal stricture or anastomosis. Am. J. Med. *20:*42–52 (Jan.) 1956.
15. Heifetz, C. J., and Senturia, H. R.: Blind intestinal pouches resulting from lateral anastomoses. Surgery *27:*673–687 (May) 1950.
16. Hertzberg, J.: Anemia associated with dilated blind segments of small intestine after side-to-side anastomoses. Acta chir. scandinav. *120:*376–379 (Jan.) 1961.
17. Holm, C. E.: Fate of sidetracked loop of ileum following lateral anastomosis for complete, benign obstruction; clinical experimental study. Surg. Gynec. & Obst. *56:*746–751 (Apr.) 1933.
18. Little, W. D., Zerfas, L. G., and Trusler, H. M.: Chronic obstruction of the small bowel. The result of two entero-enterostomies and apparently the cause of pernicious anemia. J.A.M.A. *93:*1290–1291 (Oct. 26) 1929.
19. Meulengracht, E.: Pernicious anemia in intestinal stricture (with one liver-treated case). Acta med. scandinav. *72:*231–240, 1929.
20. Panish, J. F.: Experimental blind loop steatorrhea. Gastroenterology *45:*394–399 (Sept.) 1963.
21. Siurala, M., and Kaipainen, W. J.: Intestinal megaloblastic anaemia, treated with Aureomycin and Terramycin. Acta med. scandinav. *147:*197–201, 1953.
22. Toon, R. W., and Wangensteen, O. H.: Anemia associated with blind intestinal segments and its prevention with Aureomycin. Proc. Soc. Exper. Biol. & Med. *75:*762–765 (Dec.) 1950.

Chapter Ten

TRAUMATIC LESIONS

Injuries of the small bowel may be due to nonpenetrating trauma to the abdomen or to penetrating wounds from without or within. It is estimated that one quarter to one third of all abdominal injuries involve the small bowel alone. Cottrell[2] found the small bowel injured in 10 percent of 800 cases of trauma due to falls, blasts, collisions, and so forth. With our rapidly increasing population, especially in congested urban areas, injuries of the abdomen occur frequently even in peacetime, usually as a result of an automobile accident. The diagnosis is often difficult to establish, particularly following blunt trauma to the abdomen. Laparotomy is frequently necessary to rule out such an injury.

NONPENETRATING TRAUMA

Laceration

Mechanism

Laceration of the small bowel as the result of nonpenetrating trauma usually occurs at the fixed points of the small intestine. These are at the upper jejunum near the ligament of Treitz, the lower ileum near the ileocecal valve, or at points of adhesions due to previous laparotomy or inflammation. The specific agent directly responsible for this type of injury is usually the automobile steering wheel. The bowel is crushed between the wheel and the patient's spine or pelvic bones. Occasionally the small bowel may be torn by a violent force striking the body at a tangent. Ordinarily with these injuries there is disruption of the bowel and tearing of the mesentery.

Romney[8] has reported two cases which he felt demonstrated a different mechanism. Both these patients had a small, clean perforation of the antimesenteric border with no gross damage to the adjacent bowel or mesentery. He felt that these perforations were due to the application of force to a closed loop which transmitted an explosive intraluminal wave of gas or liquid to a distant site where rupture took place.

Diagnosis

Repeated thorough examination of the abdomen by an experienced surgeon is the best means of making a diagnosis of small bowel injury after nonpenetrating trauma. Gastrointestinal trauma should always be suspected when abdominal pain, muscle spasm, and tenderness persist following severe trauma. Of these three, abdominal tenderness is the most reliable. Nausea and vomiting may or may not be present. Peritoneal irritation may be localized or generalized depending on the length of time since the injury and the degree of intraperitoneal contamination. Pain eventually becomes continuous and generalized. If it is referred to the patient's shoulder, it indicates irritation of the diaphragm by the escaped small bowel contents. A retroperitoneal rupture of the duodenum may be associated with pain that is referred to the right testicle because of irritation of the genitofemoral nerve. Peristalsis is absent or diminished. The pulse rate is increased, especially if there is extensive soiling or intraperitoneal bleeding. If hemorrhage is severe, shock may occur.

There is often evidence of intraperitoneal air by x-ray examination except in cases with duodenal rupture. Retroperitoneal air may be the only indication of duodenal rupture. Films with the patient in the upright or lateral decubitus position should always be obtained. Bleeding following duodenal injury can often be detected by gastric aspiration. A rectal examination may also reveal blood in patients with injuries of the jejunum and ileum. The leukocyte count is elevated early, but the hemoglobin and hematocrit determinations are not good indications of the degree of blood loss at this time. All patients must be observed closely for at least 72 hours with repeated examinations of the abdomen, pulse, blood pressure, respirations, hemoglobin, and white blood cell count. They should also be checked carefully for associated injuries.

Coexistent head injuries and abdominal injuries are particularly dangerous because of the patient's confusion (or coma) due to the head injury.[11] In these circumstances the signs of intraabdominal injury are likely to be masked and go unrecognized. The mortality rate in patients with blunt abdominal trauma is four times greater when associated with head injury. Wilson et al.[11] point out that abdominal rigidity and the absence of peristalsis should not be ascribed to head injury. These are signs of injury in the abdomen. If intraabdominal trauma is suspected, laparotomy should be carried out as soon as the neurologic status due to the head injury has stabilized. Abdominal paracentesis[11] or peritoneal lavage[9] are especially valuable in making the diagnosis of intraabdominal injury in comatose patients. Recently, the oral administration of diatrizoate has been suggested as a means of diagnosis of gastric or intestinal perforation.[7] It must be emphasized, however, that these and other diagnostic aids should not be allowed to delay surgery when signs of intraabdominal injury are present.

Helfrich[4] has pointed out the difficulty in making the diagnosis of perforation of the mid-small bowel. Perhaps because the contents of the bowel in this area are less irritating or less bacterially contaminated, or because the mid-small bowel is protected by the omentum, symptoms may be minimal and the diagnosis may be missed. He reported a case of small bowel perforation which was not recognized despite the fact that the patient had been hospitalized for two weeks following an injury. The patient was not aware of any abdominal discomfort, his bowel habits were normal during this time, and abdominal pain did not appear until almost three weeks following injury.

Treatment

Surgical intervention is mandatory as soon as the diagnosis of bowel injury is made. The mortality rate is proportional to the length of time between the injury and laparotomy. It is twice as high for jejunal as for ileal perforation.

The patient is prepared with intestinal decompression, antibiotics, and blood and fluid replacement. Spinal anesthesia is preferred, and a generous incision is indicated. The gastrointestinal tract and its mesentery are carefully examined. Small lacerations may be closed with a purse-string suture of silk. Larger lacerations are closed transversely. Very large lacerations and those involving the mesenteric border of the bowel are best treated by resection and end-to-end anastomosis. All ecchymotic and traumatized bowel is debrided, and the anastomosis made with healthy, actively bleeding margins of both the upper and lower loops. If there is any retroperitoneal discoloration or ecchymosis near the duodenum, this segment of the small bowel should be mobilized so that its posterior surface can be completely visualized. Cleveland and Waddell[1] reviewed 32 patients with retroperitoneal rupture of the duodenum due to nonpenetrating trauma. They were treated by direct suture, resection and end-to-end anastomosis, or duodenojejunostomy. Fourteen percent developed a fistula, but all healed. Thirty-one of the 32 patients survived.

OTHER TYPES

Perforation Due to Effort

Perforation of the small bowel due to effort is rare except in patients with an inguinal hernia.[10] In normal individuals any increase in intraabdominal pressure is immediately transmitted to the lumen of the bowel and this is balanced by the increase in pressure on the external surface of the bowel. In a patient with an incarcerated hernia, the external surface of the loop of small bowel in the hernial sac is unsupported at this point and is more likely to rupture following severe exertion. Shirer[10] reported a case in which severe effort led to rupture of a loop of small bowel that was caught in a perineal pouch. The patient had had an abdominoperineal resection for carcinoma of the rectum 18 months before. In rare instances it is associated with conditions such as periarteritis, volvulus, typhoid ulcer, and stricture of the jejunum, and also with cortisone administration.

Localized pain, swelling, and tenderness following violent effort suggest the diagnosis. This is especially true if these signs are over the sac of an inguinal hernia.

Infarction

Acute infarction of the small bowel may occur following abdominal injury. This condition is difficult to recognize and is often fatal despite treatment. It also occurs in patients in shock or congestive failure or with aortic insufficiency (Chapter Fifteen). Frequently multiple factors are present.

The classic signs of intraabdominal injury, pain, localized tenderness, and muscle guarding, are present. As peritonitis develops, the pain, tenderness, and muscle guarding become more diffuse. Fever and leukocytosis develop and peristalsis disappears. Surgical exploration of the abdomen is often the only means of establishing the diagnosis early.

The usual treatment is resection of the infarcted bowel with an end-to-end anastomosis. Recently, Frajndlich and Taylor[3] have reported a case in which, instead of resection at the time of laparotomy, intensive postoperative treatment with heparin and antibiotics was carried out. Exploration 18 hours later revealed a reversal of the pathologic process. This approach is indicated only in the patient with extensive infarction in which massive resection is incompatible with life. Laparotomy is always necessary to establish the diagnosis and the extent of the infarction.

Intramural Hematoma

Intramural hematoma of the small bowel has been reported with increasing frequency in recent years. Judd et al.[6] collected 75 cases from the literature and suggested that the lesion could be caused by minimal abdominal trauma. In their opinion the diagnosis was made usually by upper gastrointestinal study in which the pathognomonic sign was the so-called coiled spring deformity with narrowing of the bowel lumen.

Intramural hematoma of the small bowel is usually due to blunt trauma, and if it involves the duodenum or jejunum, it may lead to symptoms of high intestinal obstruction. There is a characteristic delay that varies from a few hours to several days between the onset of symptoms and the injury. Nonoperative treatment is indicated if there is no obstruction. However, if the patient does not improve or if complete obstruction develops, laparotomy should be carried out. Simple incision and drainage of the hematoma is usually sufficient, and the results are good. If the duodenum is involved, a bypass procedure may be necessary to relieve the obstruction.

PENETRATING WOUNDS

General Aspects

The mortality rate associated with penetrating wounds of the small bowel is considerably lower in civilian practice than it is on the battlefield. This is due in part to the greater proportion of stabbings or knife wounds in civilian practice which cause less extensive trauma. It is also due to the much shorter time lag between injury and operative treatment.

A good review of small bowel injury due to penetrating trauma as seen in civilian practice is found in the report by Hermann and Hubay.[5] The duodenum was involved in 2 instances, the jejunum in 21, and the ileum in 32. Twenty-four patients had solitary and 26 had multiple injuries to the small bowel. Other structures were involved in 23. Wounds of the colon were the most common associated injury. The highest mortality rate was in patients with associated injuries of the vena cava, aorta, ureter, and liver. In the majority, the injury was repaired within two hours. This was done in 30 patients by simple closure and in 19 by segmental resection. It is of interest to note that only 70 percent of these small bowel injuries were caused by external violence. Thirteen (26 percent) were produced by diagnostic or surgical procedures. The most common of these were accidental laceration of the small bowel during pelvic surgery and incision of adherent bowel when opening the abdomen. In one case a fatality resulted from a needle paracentesis in which the small bowel injury was not recognized immediately. This accident emphasizes that this diagnostic procedure is not without its serious hazards. Of the wounds from external sources, the most common were gunshot wounds and those made by sharp instruments, such as knives or icepicks. Two perforations occurred from chicken bones within the bowel. There were seven deaths, giving a mortality rate of 14 percent. Three of the deaths were directly due to the small bowel injury. All patients whose operative treatment was delayed had a complicated course. Three patients died whose repair was delayed from 20 hours to 5 days. The most important factors affecting the mortality and morbidity rates were related to delay in operative repair and the presence and nonrecognition of associated injuries to other organs.

Diagnosis

As in small bowel injury due to blunt trauma, the cardinal signs are abdominal pain, muscle guarding, and tenderness. Here, however, one also has the presence of an abdominal wound or, in the case of perforation from within, a possible history of the ingestion of a foreign body. It should not be forgotten that the small bowel, particularly the retroperitoneal duodenum, may be injured by a penetrating wound of the flank or back. Unless it can be demonstrated that the wound does not penetrate the peritoneal cavity (or the retroperitoneal duodenum), the abdomen should be explored as soon as the patient is prepared for surgery.

Treatment

These patients are prepared with intestinal intubation, antibiotics, and fluid, electrolyte, and blood replacement. A vertical incision is made near, but not through the point of injury. This must be of a sufficient length to permit examination of the entire small bowel and to exclude associated intraabdominal injury. Control of bleeding is first secured by ligation of severed vessels in the bowel, mesentery, or other abdominal viscera. Although the wounds of entrance and exit may give an approximate idea as to the course of a missile or instrument, the possibility of error (position of the body, deflection, etc.) demands a thorough examination of the entire abdomen. Close attention must be paid to the retroperitoneal duodenum. As in the case of blunt trauma to the abdomen, discoloration of the retroperitoneal tissues near the second and third portion of the duodenum is an indication for mobilization of the duodenum and visual examination of its retroperitoneal surface. This is particularly true if the wound of entrance or exit is in the flank or back. If the small bowel injury is minor it may be closed by a purse-string suture of silk. Larger wounds are closed in a transverse manner so as not to narrow the lumen of the bowel. An exception to this is a laceration of the duodenum. Here, after complete mobilization of the duodenum and head of the pancreas, the laceration is often best closed longitudinally. Transverse closure of a large laceration in the duodenum is apt to produce tension at the suture line. If there are several perforations of the small bowel closely grouped together, resection of this segment of bowel followed by an end-to-end anastomosis is indicated. Large lacerations of the small bowel, especially when the mesenteric border is involved, are also best treated by resection and end-to-end anastomosis. The mesenteric defect is closed, and associated injuries are treated as indicated. The peritoneal cavity is washed with copious amounts of saline, and all contaminated fluid is aspirated. Any denuded surface of the bowel is peritonealized as completely as possible, since small bowel obstruction may follow small bowel injury. Unless there are associated injuries, the peritoneal cavity is closed without drainage. The incision is also irrigated with saline, since postoperative wound infections are common in these patients.

SUMMARY

The small bowel is the most frequently injured abdominal organ. In civilian life, nonpenetrating trauma is more common and usually more serious than are penetrating wounds of the small bowel. The former type is due primarily to the large number of automobile accidents that occur. Abdominal tenderness and the absence of peristalsis are valuable signs of intraabdominal injury. The mortality rate increases rapidly with delay in operative treatment. Repeated thorough examination of the abdomen by an experienced surgeon is the most effective means of making the diagnosis of blunt, nonpenetrating trauma.

Unless it can be demonstrated that an external wound of the abdomen does not penetrate the peritoneal cavity, the abdomen should be explored as soon as the patient can be prepared for surgery. This applies to wounds of the flank or back as well as the anterior abdominal wall. The abdominal exploration should be carefully and methodically done, not forgetting the retroperitoneal duodenum. The most important factor that increases the mortality rate in a patient with a penetrating wound of the small bowel is delay in operative repair.

REFERENCES

1. Cleveland, H. C., and Waddell, W. R.: Retroperitoneal rupture of the duodenum due to nonpenetrating trauma. S. Clin. North America *43:*413–431 (Apr.) 1963.
2. Cottrell, J. C.: Nonperforative trauma to abdomen. Arch. Surg. *68:*241–251 (Feb.) 1954.
3. Frajndlich, D., and Taylor, R. L.: Infarction of the small bowel. J.A.M.A. *189:*327–328 (July 27) 1964.
4. Helfrich, R. B.: Difficulty in diagnosing perforation of mid-small bowel. Hawaii M. J. *20:*333–334 (Mar.-Apr.) 1961.
5. Hermann, R. E., and Hubay, C. A.: Perforating injury of the small intestine. Mechanisms of injury and factors affecting mortality. Arch. Surg. *88:*290–294 (Feb.) 1964.
6. Judd, D. R., Taybi, H., and King, H.: Intramural hematoma of the small bowel; a report of two cases and a review of the literature. Arch. Surg. *89:*527–535 (Sept.) 1964.
7. McCraw, J., McLeod, R., McDonald, W., et al.: A urine precipitation test for intestinal perforation. Arch. Surg. *91:*248–252 (Aug.) 1965.
8. Romney, D.: Perforation of bowel by nonpenetrating trauma. Northwest Med. *61:*404–405 (May) 1962.
9. Root, H. D., Hauser, C. W., McKinley, C. R., et al.: Diagnostic peritoneal lavage. Surgery *57:*633–637 (May) 1965.
10. Shirer, W. C.: Rupture of small bowel due to effort after abdominoperineal excision of rectum. Brit. J. Surg. *49:*689–690 (May) 1962.
11. Wilson, C. B., Vidrine, A. J., and Rives, J. D.: Unrecognized abdominal trauma in patients with head injuries. Ann. Surg. *161:*608–613 (Apr.) 1965.

Chapter Eleven

RADIATION ENTERITIS

Another type of injury to the small bowel that is of clinical importance is that resulting from radiation, usually secondary to the treatment of gynecologic cancer. Rosen and Shapiro,[4] have recently reviewed this problem and estimate that radiation proctitis occurs in 50 to 100 percent and radiation enteritis in 1 to 9 percent of patients undergoing radiation treatment for malignancy of the pelvic organs. Since in Ontario alone 985 new patients with gynecologic cancer are registered every year, they point out that a significant number of women will be found to be suffering from radiation injury to the small bowel. The incidence of actinic enteritis of the small bowel serious enough to require surgical treatment is of course smaller than that of the less severe forms; yet series of 34,[5] 5,[3] and 6[2] patients who received surgical treatment are reported in the literature.

Severe symptoms resulting from an acute inflammatory reaction in the bowel wall may occur within a few months after treatment. On the other hand, the first indication of radiation damage may be a sudden perforation of the small intestine a year or more after treatment. A great danger arises when symptoms of obstruction from radiation injury of the small bowel occur months or years after radiation treatment for malignant disease. Most likely, the symptoms then are attributed to recurrent carcinoma of the pelvis, and the patient is treated conservatively. Schier et al.[5] have reported a range of intervals of from 3 months to 25 years from the initial radiation treatment to the appearance of the first symptoms. In 32 percent of cases, symptoms developed within the first year.

PATHOLOGY

The mucosa of the intestinal tract contains cells which are extremely sensitive to irradiation.[1] Within 24 hours of exposure, the mucosa and

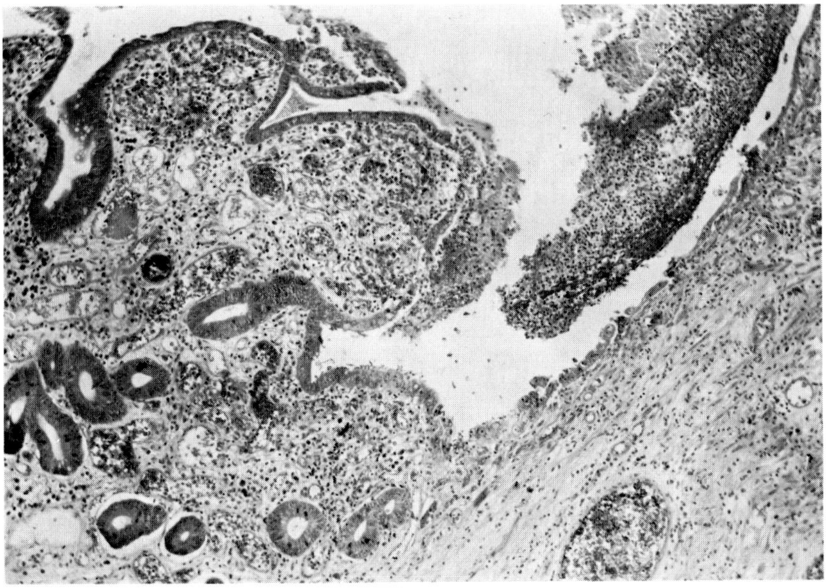

Figure 11–1. Photomicrograph of actinic ulcer of small intestine showing beginning regeneration.

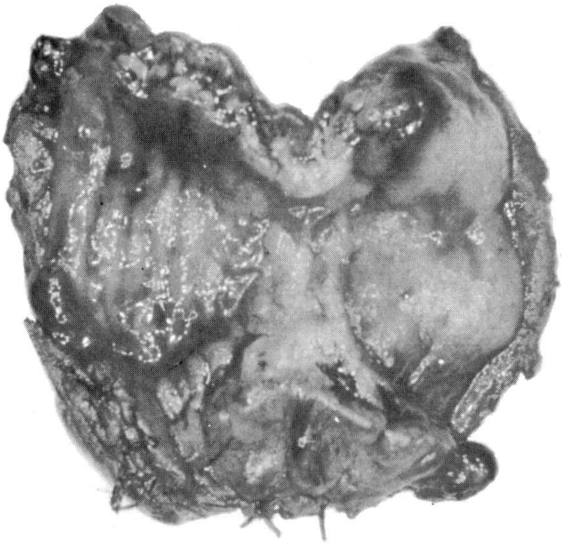

Figure 11–2. Radiation ulcer of small intestine causing contraction of the wall and stenosis of the lumen.

submucosa show edema and cell degeneration. When the edema subsides, atrophy occurs followed by regeneration. Complications occur when a chronic ulcer develops at the site of injury. In the more serious cases the primary injury is to the blood vessels in the intestinal wall, leading to endarteritis, thrombosis, and subsequent infarction. The mucosa ulcerates, leaving single or multiple irregular superficial erosions that often progress to deep, punched-out, discrete ulcers with a ragged, grayish base and sharp margins (Fig. 11–1). The ulcer of the small bowel may then perforate into the peritoneal cavity, producing generalized peritonitis. At other times a fistula or abscess may form between the small bowel and contiguous organs. The end result of these inflammatory lesions may be cicatricial stenosis of the intestine producing the common complication, obstruction (Fig. 11–2).

At operation, the following findings are typical: the peritoneum is thickened and the bowel grayish-white, mottled, and edematous with areas of telangiectasis. Ascites may be present. In spite of its thickened, hoselike appearance, the bowel is often friable, and care must be taken in freeing any adhesions which are present.

CLINICAL ASPECTS

Radiation injury of the small bowel often causes rectal bleeding, cramps, and diarrhea when the treatment is nearly completed, just as is seen in radiation proctitis. These symptoms usually subside with the completion of therapy. When they persist for several months following therapy, further symptoms from radiation injury may be expected.

Although small bowel injury is much less common than rectal injury, it is likely to be more serious in its consequences. Established actinic enteritis is marked by abdominal pain, vomiting, alternating constipation and diarrhea, and rectal bleeding.[3, 5] The abdominal pain is usually sharp and cramping and relieved by vomiting. Physical examination often discloses actinodermatitis of the lower abdomen. At times a mass is palpable in the abdomen or pelvis and represents matted loops of bowel. A history of radiation therapy for pelvic carcinoma should be ascertained in any patient with symptoms of small bowel obstruction.

REPORT OF A CASE

A 60-year-old woman had been given primary therapy of 9,000 R by a 2,000,000-volt x-ray unit for carcinoma of the cervix, stage 3. Seventeen months after completion of therapy, abdominal pain, melena, diarrhea, vomiting, and weight loss developed. A barium enema showed narrowing of the rectum. Proctitis was present at the 4-inch level. A mass had previously been noted on rectal examination six months after completion of therapy and was still palpable at the time of the onset of symptoms. The proctitis subsided, but symptoms of partial intestinal obstruction continued for three years. She was admitted to the hospital three and one half years after radiation treatment and died 24 hours after admission. Autopsy revealed no residual tumor. Death was caused by generalized peritonitis secondary to radiation necrosis of the ileum with perforation.

Comment. The delayed symptoms of nausea, weight loss, and abdominal pain were not caused by radiation proctitis or by recurrence of the carcinoma of the cervix. If a laparotomy had been performed when the symptoms of low-grade obstruction developed, the patient probably would have survived. Five patients in our group of 41 died as a direct result of radiation injury to the small intestine,[3] and in 2 patients no malignant disease was found at autopsy. Radiation injury to the terminal ileum may occur in the absence of any previous surgery leading to fixation of the small bowel in the pelvis.[3]

SURGICAL TREATMENT AND RESULTS

Surgical treatment is necessary for any of the complications of actinic enteritis. These are obstruction, fistula, abscess formation, or free perforation, which occur in that order of frequency. If symptoms of obstruction persist in a patient with a history of pelvic irradiation, surgical intervention should be considered seriously. Surgery is also necessary when an enterovesical or enterovaginal fistula develops. Although a sidetracking anastomosis between healthy loops of bowel may be necessary in a poor-risk patient, resection of the diseased bowel is the treatment of choice. It enables one to rule out recurrent carcinoma or other similar lesions such as regional enteritis. In addition the end results are better. Death from hemorrhage in the sidetracked bowel has been reported.[5] The abrupt onset of peritonitis in any patient who has received radiation therapy of the pelvis is of course an indication for immediate laparotomy.

It is important to make certain that one is using healthy bowel for the anastomosis. Normal appearing bowel close to that which contains telangiectasis obviously due to radiation may not be completely normal in its ability to form a solid union. Frozen section examination of the cut margin may be of help in ruling out radiation injury, but the safest course is to allow an ample margin (2 to 3 inches) of apparently normal bowel on either side of the lesion. Although we have not used it, the insertion of a proximal enterostomy tube as an additional safety factor should be considered. When no healthy distal ileum remains, the anastomosis is made between the terminal portion of normal small bowel and the ascending colon. If peritonitis is present, a modified Mikulicz resection offers a way out of a difficult situation. In one report, leakage occurred in 2 of 39 anastomoses.[5]

The mortality of patients treated for advanced small bowel actinic enteritis is high. In one series of 34 patients requiring surgery, 5 patients died in the postoperative period.[5] In another series of 13, 4 died postoperatively.[6]

CONCLUSIONS

Serious injury to the small bowel, usually the ileum, can occur as a result of irradiation therapy to the pelvis, particularly in patients with carcinoma of the cervix. The interval between the radiation and the onset of symptoms may be months or many years. A patient with signs of persistent small bowel obstruction and a history of radiation therapy to the pelvis requires surgical treatment before perforation and peritonitis develop. The treatment of choice is resection with anastomosis of the distal and proximal uninjured small bowel.

REFERENCES

1. Anderson, W. C. A.: Pathology. Ed. 3. St. Louis, Mo., C. V. Mosby Co., 1957.
2. Aune, E. F., and White, B. V.: Gastrointestinal complications of irradiation for carcinoma of uterine cervix. J.A.M.A. *147:*831–834 (Oct. 27) 1951.
3. Colcock, B. P., and Hume, A.: Radiation injury to the sigmoid and rectum. Surg. Gynec. & Obst. *108:*306–312 (Mar.) 1959.
4. Rosen, I. B., and Shapiro, B. J.: Radiation enteropathy of the small bowel. Canad. M. A. J. *91:*681–688 (Sept. 26) 1964.
5. Schier, J., Symmonds, R. E., and Dahlin, D. C.: Clinicopathologic aspects of actinic enteritis. Surg. Gynec. & Obst. *119:*1019–1025 (Nov.) 1964.
6. White, W. C., and Finn, F. W.: Late complications following irradiation of pelvic viscera. Am. J. Obst. & Gynec. *62:*65–74 (July) 1951.

Chapter Twelve

FISTULAS

Fistulas of the small intestine are a major catastrophy of surgical practice. The results of their treatment vary in the literature (Table 12–1) from a 17 percent mortality for mesenteric small bowel fistulas[17] to a 67 percent mortality for lateral duodenal fistulas.[7] Further compounding this tragedy is the observation that approximately 70 percent are due to a technical error of the surgeon and thus follow an operative procedure.[7]

The treatment of small bowel fistulas has many facets based at times on fact, at times on experience and judgment, and at other times on controversy. Before further consideration of the subject can be given, however, certain facts relative to the classification and peculiarities of various fistulas must be known. Table 12–2 shows a working classification of small bowel fistulas based on their location, their volume flow, and their drainage pattern. In this chapter, we will limit our discussion (as have most authors) to a consideration of duodenal, jejunal, and ileal fistulas that drain a large volume externally (at least 100 cc. per day). The variations in results and opinions regarding treatment expressed in the literature are in some measure due to the inclusion in some series of low flow or internal fistulas of a less serious prognosis.

CAUSE AND PREVENTION

The cause of small intestinal fistulas can be traced in most cases to operative injury and technical difficulties (Table 12–3). Thus, Edmunds et al.[7] found 67 percent to be due to technical failure including anastomotic leak, surgical injury, and gross surgical error. When just jejunal and ileal fistulas are considered, 22 of 23 fistulas could be traced to surgical misadventure.[17]

In view of the poor results and high mortality in the treatment of small bowel fistulas, their prevention assumes major importance and is based on

Table 12-1. Mortality (Percent) of Small Intestinal Fistulas

AUTHOR	SITE UNSPECIFIED	DUODENUM *End*	*Both*	*Lateral*	MESENTERIC BOWEL *Jejunum*	*Both*	*Ileum*
Bowlin et al.[3]	33	13		54			
Braasch and Nickerson[4]		17		43	43		18
Chapman et al.[5]			57			65	
Edmunds et al.[7]	54	52		67			
West et al.[17]			31			17	

Table 12-2. Classification of Small Intestinal Fistulas

- Anatomic
  - Duodenal
    - End
    - Side
  - Jejunal—ileal
    - High
    - Low
- Flow
  - High volume (100 cc./day)
  - Low volume
- Drainage pattern
  - External (skin, vagina, perineum)
  - Internal

Table 12-3. Etiology of Small Intestinal Fistulas

	EDMUNDS ET AL.[7] 1960		WEST ET AL.[17] 1961 (*jejunal and ileal*)	
Surgical complication	33		22	
Anastomosis failure		19		7
Operative injury		11		9
Prolapse of bowel into dehiscence				5
Gross surgical error		3		
Wire mesh perforate bowel				1
Obstruction	5		1	
Inflammatory disease	2			
Carcinoma	3			
Trauma	3			

the use of a careful surgical technique. Anastomoses should have a more than adequate blood supply; suture lines should be watertight; there should be no tension on anastomoses or closures; and care must be exercised in the closure of the abdominal wall so that loops of intestine are not included in the suture. The management of the duodenal stump deserves special care in the application of these precautions.

GENERAL MANAGEMENT

The general management of fistulas of the small intestine is best discussed under the headings of nutrition and hydration, skin care, treatment and prevention of infection, various miscellaneous points, and the major decision of the indication for surgical attack (Table 12–4).

NUTRITION AND HYDRATION

Patients with high-flow fistulas present major problems in fluid and electrolyte management. Replacement of lost water, sodium, chloride, and potassium is vital. For long-term fistulas attention must also be given to magnesium replacement. For this reason quantitative collection of fluid losses is important. The results of replacement of these elements should be monitored by blood electrolyte determinations and body weight observations. Replacement may be in the form of intravenous fluids, or the recovered fluid

Table 12–4. Supportive Treatment for Small Intestinal Fistulas

- Nutrition and hydration
  - Feed
    - Oral (with low fistulas)
    - Tube (with low fistulas)
    - Jejunostomy (proximal fistulas)
  - Water, electrolytes, blood intravenously
  - Protein and fat intravenously
- Skin care
  - Suction
  - Skin protection
  - Stryker frame
- Control infection
  - Antibiotics
  - Abscesses—recognize and drain
- Miscellaneous
  - Slow diarrhea
  - Low-residue diet for distal fistulas
  - Prevent and treat the complications
    - Hemorrhage
    - Phlebitis and embolism
    - Pancreatitis

Table 12-5. Formula Suitable for Blendorization and Use With Barron Pump*

Boiled potato	1 cup		
Cooked cereal	2 cups		
Floating island base	16 oz.		
Strained baby meat (chicken and beef)	4 cans		
Sustagen powder	$2\frac{1}{2}$ cups		
Lactose	$\frac{1}{4}$ cup		
Water	5 cups		
	1300 cc.	containing 1.3 calories/cc.	
		carbohydrate	343 gm.
		fat	84 gm.
		protein	175 gm.

* Adapted from Warren, K. W., et al.: Dis. Colon & Rectum *8*:26 (Jan.-Feb.) 1965.

may be returned to the patient by jejunostomy or long nasal tube, the end of which is distal to the fistula. In addition to the replacement of lost fluid and electrolytes, tube feeding mixtures should be given with the aid of a food pump as designed by Barron.[2] With the use of this pump, more than 2000 calories a day can be delivered to the uninvolved intestine for absorption. The great advantage of such a pump is that a more concentrated mixture can be reliably administered through a smaller nonirritating tube with less chance of diarrhea. Table 12–5 gives the contents of a 1300 cc. tube feeding mixture which is suitable for use with the pump and which provides 1690 calories and 175 gm. of protein.

Of less efficiency is the administration of calories and protein by the intravenous route in the form of albumin and protein and fat hydrolysates. The use of blood transfusions when indicated should not be neglected.

SKIN CARE

The care of the skin around the fistula and the collection of lost fluid is of understandable importance, and there are many techniques for accomplishing these ends. The use of wound suction is one method of fluid collection valuable especially in more proximal fistulas with liquid discharge. A large size catheter with additional holes should be placed adjacent to the fistula but not penetrating the defect in the bowel. A vent may be provided by inserting a needle into the catheter at skin level. Another method for fluid collection and skin protection in fistulas with relatively intact skin edges is the application of a Fazio ileostomy bag to the opening. In cases in which neither of these methods is applicable, the use of a Stryker frame with dependent drainage into a collecting basin under the prone patient has at times succeeded.

A large number of creams, ointments, and powders have been used to protect the surrounding skin from irritation. These include zinc oxide ointment, aluminum paste, vitamin A and D ointment, and many others. Our preference is for a diatomaceous earth (fullers' earth), which dries the skin and has great protective powers.

INFECTION CONTROL

The third major area of importance in the supportive treatment of patients with small bowel fistulas is the control of sepsis. Abscesses, peritonitis, and septicemia frequently accompany fistulas and must be combated with the appropriate antibotics and with the timely drainage of purulent collections. Subphrenic, subhepatic, and pelvic abscesses must be repeatedly looked for in any patient with fever and a fistula.

MISCELLANEOUS CONSIDERATIONS

Gastric suction probably does little to influence the healing even of duodenal fistulas. It removes fluid and electrolytes, part of which might not be lost in the fistulous drainage. In cases of distal small bowel fistulas, a low-residue diet and measures to slow diarrhea seem to have merit and could cut down on calorie, fluid, and electrolyte losses.

Awareness of the commoner complications of fistulas, hemorrhage and pulmonary embolism, is important. The prevention of phlebitis is essential in these chronically ill patients.

INDICATIONS FOR OPERATION

The place and the timing of operative intervention for small intestinal fistulas has aroused controversy in the surgical literature. There is agreement that surgical treatment should be undertaken for any fistula that does not close with optimum conservative management. Chapman et al.[5] assign more importance to the nutritional features of fistula management and use surgical closure as a last resort. Opposed are Edmunds et al.[7] who recommend surgical attack one to three weeks after the onset of the fistula and point out the dangers of deterioration of the patient with procrastination and excessive reliance on conservative measures. It seems logical to delay surgical treatment at least while the patient is gaining in nutrition and the fluid spaces are being restored to normal. Surgical attack on recent duodenal fistulas holds little promise of success, and operative intervention should be delayed for a matter of months. In cases of high-flow jejunal and ileal fistulas, it is unlikely that conservative management will be successful, and operative attack is recommended at a relatively early date.

At times, small bowel fistulas are associated with obstruction of the intestine distal to the fistula. It is important that such a condition be corrected at the time of any contemplated surgical repair, and, in fact, obstruction is a definite indication for early operative intervention.

OPERATIVE PROCEDURES

The general operative approaches to the treatment of small intestinal fistulas can be classified into definitive and nondefinitive procedures (Table 12–6).

NONDEFINITIVE PROCEDURES

It is obvious from the large number of procedures available for the treatment of each case and from the high mortality of small bowel fistulas that none of the recommended procedures is entirely satisfactory. Feeding jejunostomy is of use only with fistulas proximal to the jejunostomy site. Bypass procedures are generally not effective. Incomplete bypass by side-to-side anastomosis is merely a surgical exercise and sidetracks only a small proportion of the succus entericus. Bypass by end-to-side anastomosis with turn-in of the distal bowel is more effective, but still does not prevent loss through the fistula by retrograde flow through the efferent loop. In the case of duodenal fistulas, pyloric exclusion, accomplished by resection of the antrum, duodenal closure, vagotomy, and gastrojejunostomy, is effective in some cases in decreasing fluid loss. If reflux through the afferent loop is minimal, oral feeding might be permitted following this procedure.

The general inadvisability of bypass procedures is reflected in the poor results of nine failures in nine operations reported by Edmunds et al.[7] and three failures in four operations reported by Chapman et al.[5]

Table 12–6. Operative Procedures for Small Bowel Fistulas

Nondefinitive operations
Feeding jejunostomy
Bypass procedures
Complete pyloric exclusion (duodenal)
Definitive operations
Suture closure
Resection and anastomosis
Anastomosis to fistula (duodenal fistulas)
Side-to-side anastomosis
Roux-Y anastomosis
Patch closure (duodenal fistulas)
Complete exclusion

DEFINITIVE PROCEDURES

Generally, direct suture of fistulous openings can be done only under certain circumstances in which the edge of the bowel is not friable and the opening in the bowel is small. Ordinarily the procedure of choice is resection of the involved bowel and anastomosis. In the special circumstance in which the operator elects to approach a jejunal or ileal fistula through the abdomen at a distance from the fistula, the procedure of Keyes and Middleman[10] and of Harbison[8] of complete exclusion of the fistula is of value (Fig. 12–1). In this procedure the bowel proximal and distal to the fistula is divided, and an anastomosis is accomplished between the proximal and distal bowel. The fistulous loop may then be excised, or the ends may be oversewn or exteriorized. Of help is the preoperative placement of a long intestinal tube proximally and Foley catheters through the fistula into the afferent and efferent loops to aid in identification of the proximal, distal, and fistulous bowel at surgery.

The use of jejunal patch closure or side-to-side or Roux-Y anastomosis to close fistulas is particularly applicable to duodenal fistulas and will be considered later.

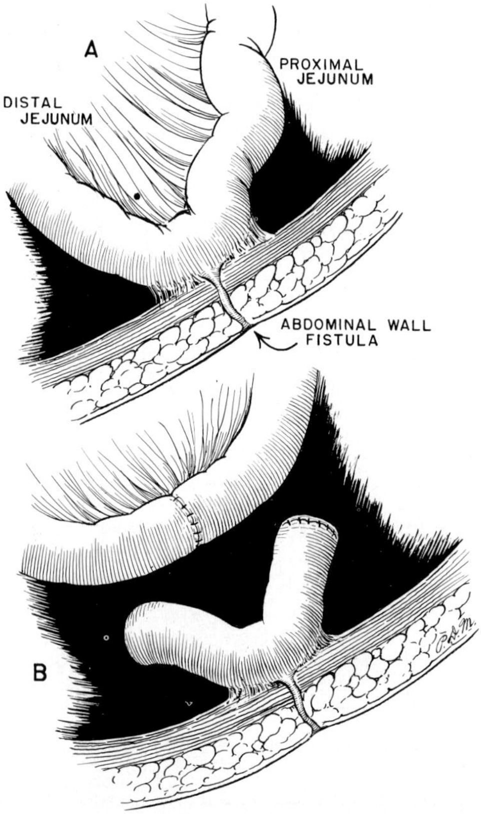

Figure 12–1. Complete exclusion of small bowel fistula by disconnection and anastomosis.

The results obtained in the management of small intestinal fistulas depend in large part on the nutritional state of the patient and the volume flow through the fistula. In a study of 25 high-output fistulas, 11 cases were optimal nutritionally at the time of treatment and only two failed to be controlled.[5] Conversely in 14 cases who were suboptimal nutritionally, 13 fistula closures failed and there were 13 fatalities. This observation is borne out by our study of 73 small intestinal fistulas in which there was a high degree of correlation between death and high output and malnutrition.[4]

SPECIFIC FISTULAS

Because of special characteristics of fistulas in various parts of the small intestine, it is advantageous to consider duodenal, jejunal and high ileal, and low ileal fistulas separately.

DUODENAL FISTULAS

Duodenal fistulas are either end (stump) fistulas or side fistulas. The latter are in continuity with the gastrointestinal tract, are generally higher-flow fistulas, and have a higher mortality, about 50 percent.[3, 4, 7] Leakage from the closed duodenal stump, the most serious complication of gastric resection, occurs following approximately 3 percent of gastric resections.[13] The mortality of this complication varies in reported series of cases from 13 to 52 percent (Table 12–1).

Cause

As a rule, more than one factor is involved in a perforation of a duodenal stump. General causes such as malnutrition, anemia, or carcinoma may play a part, but local causes are predominant. An extensive dissection may lead to devitalization of an area of duodenum at the line of closure. Inadequate inversion, tension on the suture line, or postoperative pancreatitis may result in a blowout of a duodenal stump. The most frequent local causes are an acute inflammatory reaction in the duodenal wall due to a duodenal ulcer and the development of increased intraluminal pressure in the afferent loop following a gastrojejunal anastomosis.

Prevention

By far the most important aspect of this problem is its prevention. Certain technical steps are of value when there is very little posterior duodenal wall left to invert following gastric resection. This is often true with a posterior wall ulcer that has perforated against the pancreas. None of the remaining posterior wall should be lost by crushing it with a clamp or destroying it with cautery. In most patients, a careful dissection of the posterior wall below the ulcer will permit the insertion of at least one row of interrupted silk sutures to close the duodenum. If the dissection is not carried down the medial side of the duodenum for more than a quarter of an inch, the likelihood of injury to the common bile duct or the duct of Wirsung is small. If there is any doubt about the location of the common bile duct, it should be exposed and intubated. After closure, the suture line is covered by the mesentery surrounding the ligated right gastric artery above and the ligated right gastroepiploic artery below. If a single row of interrupted, nonabsorbable sutures uniting duodenum to duodenum cannot be placed, the redundant lateral wall of the duodenum may be sutured to the lower edge of the ulcer base by interrupted silk sutures. This, in turn, is covered by adjacent omentum or mesentery. Special types of suture may be employed in this difficult situation as suggested by Copello.[6] All patients in whom the duodenal closure has been difficult should have drains placed to Morison's pouch.

The problem of a difficult duodenal closure can be avoided by using a two-stage procedure. The first stage, a gastric resection, is carried out leaving a segment of antrum which is closed. The retained antrum should be removed within six to eight weeks if one is to avoid the development of a stomal ulcer. This is true even though a vagotomy has also been done. This has the disadvantage of being a two-stage procedure, and it may be that even in six to eight weeks the ulcer will still be adherent to the pancreas and closure of the duodenal stump may still be difficult.

The Bancroft procedure has been used to meet this problem and at the same time avoid a second operation. The antrum is divided proximal to the duodenum, and the cause of recurrent ulceration, the antral mucosa, is removed from the distal gastric stump. Following this, the muscularis and serosa of the gastric stump are inverted. This carries the risk that a closed loop may be produced between an area of stenosis produced by the ulcer and the closed antrum. Leakage from the closed antrum has occurred with serious consequences.

A Roux-Y duodenojejunostomy has been suggested by Barnett.[1] The Roux-Y loop of jejunum is sutured to the duodenum over the open or partially closed stump. Many inverting sutures can be used since it is not necessary to avoid narrowing the lumen of either segment.

In recent years, a planned, duodenal fistula (tube duodenostomy) has had widespread use as an answer to this problem.[15] Although the mortality associated with this procedure is low, it is not without its hazards as Robertson[14] has pointed out. The hospital stay of the patient is considerably prolonged, although it may well be shorter than it would have been had a duodenal leak developed. Fluid and electrolyte replacement is a problem unless a jejunostomy is carried out. Severe hemorrhage can occur, since all the alkaline bile and duodenal contents bypass the gastrojejunal anastomosis, and an anastomotic ulcer may develop very quickly. If a tube duodenostomy is used, the advice of those who have had the most experience with its use

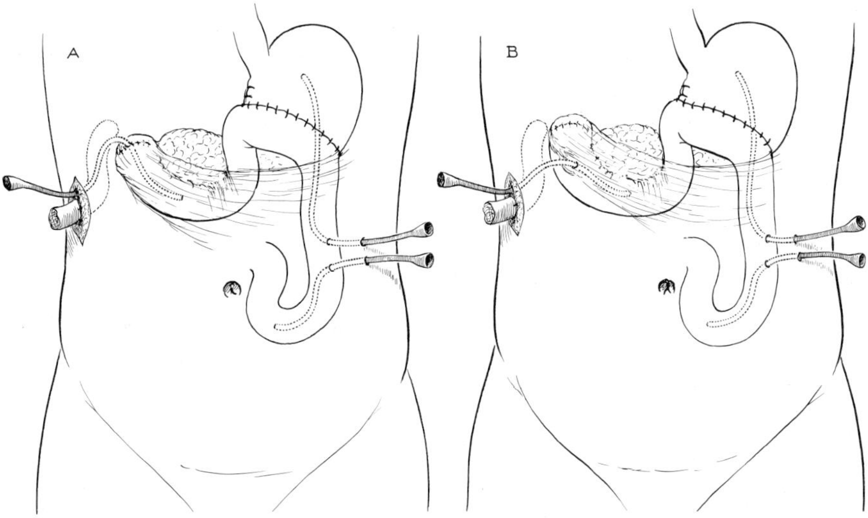

Figure 12–2. Tube duodenostomy with double jejunostomy in the management of the difficult duodenal stump. *A,* Original procedure; *B,* modification.

should be followed closely. In the original procedure, the end of the duodenum was closed about a catheter and a drain inserted down to this area. A double jejunostomy is established 6 to 8 inches below the gastrojejunal anastomosis. One catheter is placed proximally into the stomach and the other well down into the distal jejunum (Fig. 12–2*A*). A modification of this procedure (not always applicable) consists of placing a catheter in the side of the duodenum following closure of the open end (Fig. 12–2*B*). This whistle-tip catheter should be no larger than a No. 12 or 14 French, and is fixed in place by two catgut, purse-string sutures, the first of which transfixes the catheter. If a large amount of duodenal drainage develops from the duodenal tube, it is connected to the distal jejunostomy tube after peristalsis has returned. The duodenal drain is removed on the eighth postoperative day, the duodenal catheter on the eleventh, and the jejunostomy tube or tubes on the twelfth postoperative day.

It is our opinion that the best way to manage the problem of a difficult duodenal stump closure is to avoid it completely. This can be done by the use of a reasonably good operative procedure for duodenal ulcer, namely, vagotomy and posterior gastroenterostomy. Although this procedure may not be the best operation for all patients with a duodenal ulcer, we think it is the best operation for the patient whose duodenum cannot be closed securely. It is important to remember that the surgeon must make this decision before he opens the duodenum.

The prevention of lateral duodenal fistulas generally involves a secure closure of a duodenotomy incision. We believe a longitudinal closure with care not to obstruct the lumen is safer than a transverse closure.

Table 12–7. Results of Conservative Treatment of Duodenal Fistulas

Author	End fistulas		Side fistulas	
	Total Cases	*Closed Cases*	*Total Cases*	*Closed Cases*
Bowlin et al.[3]	8	7	10	5
West et al.[17]	12	10	4	2

Treatment

In general, duodenal fistulas should be managed conservatively with suction and a feeding jejunostomy. Table 12–7 shows representative results of conservative management. As mentioned previously, the procedure of duodenal exclusion is at times warranted to cut down the volume of flow from the fistula. Operative attack directly on the fistula has been used only months after the onset of the fistula and, under these circumstances, cure has been accomplished in 7 of 8 lateral fistulas and 4 of 8 stump fistulas reviewed in the literature up to 1959.[7] Table 12–8 shows our results with surgical closures of 10 end duodenal fistulas and 12 side fistulas. Definitive closure of the end fistulas was delayed an average of 23 weeks after the onset of the fistula and under these conditions was successful in 8 of 10 cases.

Because of the high overall mortality in the treatment of duodenal fistulas, two new approaches to the problem have been reported. In one the usefulness of an anastomosis between the fistula and a simple or a Roux-Y loop of jejunum has been demonstrated in animal investigation.[9] Two other groups of investigators have reported the use of a patch technique wherein the serosa of a loop of jejunum has been used to close defects of the duodenum in dogs.[11, 18] These surgeons reported enough encouragement with these techniques to indicate a clinical trial.

Jejunal and Proximal Ileal Fistulas

Jejunal and proximal ileal fistulas usually should be managed conservatively unless they are of high flow. With high-volume fistulas, conservative management should be continued only long enough to improve the patient's

Table 12–8. Results of Definitive Surgical Closure of End and Lateral Duodenal Fistulas*

Type	Total cases	Death	Successful closure
End fistula	10	1	8
Side fistula	12	5	5

* From Braasch, J. W., and Nickerson, W. R.: The management of small intestinal fistulas. In preparation.

general condition in preparation for operative repair. Ordinarily resection and anastomosis or complete exclusion and anastomosis are the procedures of choice. A mortality of about 40 percent (Table 12–1) has been reported with significant fistulas, although Edmunds et al.[7] have reported cures in 16 of 17 cases of high-flow fistulas treated by primary resection with or without preliminary bypass.

DISTAL ILEAL FISTULAS

Lower ileal fistulas lend themselves to conservative management and can be expected to close spontaneously in a much higher proportion than proximal fistulas.[12] Their flow volume is less, and malnutrition is uncommon because of the efficiency for absorption of a normal proximal bowel. If, however, they persist beyond four to six weeks, direct surgical closure is indicated.

REFERENCES

1. Barnett, W. O.: Investigations regarding the management of the duodenal stump. Surg. Gynec. & Obst. *113:*197–204 (Aug.) 1961.
2. Barron, J.: Tube feeding of postoperative patients. S. Clin. North America *39:*1481–1491 (Dec.) 1959.
3. Bowlin, J. W., Hardy, J. O., and Conn, J. H.: External alimentary fistulas. Analysis of 79 cases with notes on management. Am. J. Surg. *103:*6–14 (Jan.) 1962.
4. Braasch, J. W., and Nickerson, W. R.: The management of small intestinal fistulas. In preparation.
5. Chapman, R., Foran, R., and Dunphy, J. E.: Management of intestinal fistulas. Am. J. Surg. *108:*157–164 (Aug.) 1964.
6. Copello, A. J.: Closure of the duodenal stump in difficult cases. Surgery *54:*713–715 (Nov.) 1963.
7. Edmunds, L. H., Jr., Williams, G. M., and Welch, C. E.: External fistulas arising from the gastrointestinal tract. Ann. Surg. *152:*445–471 (Sept.) 1960.
8. Harbison, S. P.: The principle of complete exclusion in fistulas of the small intestine. Surgery *28:*384–392 (Aug.) 1950.
9. Jones, S. A., and Joergenson, E. J.: Closure of duodenal wall defects. Surgery *53:*438–442 (Apr.) 1963.
10. Keyes, E. L., and Middleman, I. C.: Treatment of fistula and obstruction of the small intestine by complete exclusion. Surg. Gynec. & Obst. *72:*237–243 (Feb.) 1941.
11. Kobald, E. E., and Thal, A. P.: A simple method for the management of experimental wounds of the duodenum. Surg. Gynec. & Obst. *116:*340–344 (Mar.) 1963.
12. Lichtman, A. L., and McDonald, J. R.: Fecal fistula. Surg. Gynec. & Obst. *78:*449–470 (May) 1944.
13. Pearce, C. W., Jordan, G. L., Jr., and DeBakey, M. E.: Intra-abdominal complications following distal subtotal gastrectomy for benign gastroduodenal ulceration. Surgery *42:*447–461 (Sept.) 1957.
14. Robertson, H. R.: The duodenal stump. Surg. Gynec. & Obst. *101:*636–637 (Nov.) 1955.
15. Rodkey, G. V., and Welch, C. E.: Duodenal decompression in gastrectomy. Further experiences with duodenostomy. New England J. Med. *262:*498–501 (Mar. 10) 1960.
16. Warren, K. W., Frederick, P. L., and Zomorodian, A. A.: Restoration and maintenance of metabolic balance during the preoperative and postoperative phases by artificial feeding in the debilitated patient. Dis. Colon & Rectum *8:*23–29 (Jan.-Feb.) 1965.
17. West, J. P., Ring, E. M., Miller, R. E., et al.: A study of causes and treatment of external postoperative intestinal fistulas. Surg. Gynec. & Obst. *113:*490–496 (Oct.) 1961.
18. Wolfman, E. F., Jr., Trevino, G., Heaps, D. K., et al.: An operative technique for the management of acute and chronic lateral duodenal fistulas. Ann. Surg. *159:*563–569 (Apr.) 1964.

Chapter Thirteen

ENTEROSTOMY

Enterostomy has assumed increasing importance in the surgeon's armamentarium in recent years. Duodenostomy, jejunostomy, and ileostomy, although indicated by different circumstances, can be the determining factor in the survival of the patient and so deserve close scrutiny.

Duodenostomy has been discussed in another chapter (Chapter Twelve, Fistulas) and will not be covered here, but a consideration of jejunostomy and ileostomy follows.

JEJUNOSTOMY

Indications

The usual indication for a high jejunostomy is the need for feeding a malnourished patient, either preliminary to or following a major operative procedure. In addition it may become a lifesaving measure when large volumes of fistulous drainage must be returned to the patient or replaced. Occasionally it is used to decompress the small bowel proximal to the point of a major resection or the stomach following gastric resection and a gastrojejunostomy. Rarely today, a low jejunostomy is carried out in patients with adynamic ileus when intubation and all other methods have failed to relieve the distention.

Technique

When employed for feeding or to decompress the stomach, the jejunostomy is established through a stab wound in the left upper quadrant near the ligament of Treitz. Usually one of two methods is used. In the case of a Stamm enterostomy, a loop of proximal jejunum is selected, sufficient to reach from the ligament of Treitz to the anterior abdominal wall. The proximal and distal ends are identified, the contents of a 3- to 4-inch loop are stripped, and occluding clamps are applied above and below. Two concentric purse-string sutures are placed in the antimesenteric border. Usually, a No. 16 French catheter is used, which is passed down the bowel for approximately 15 to 20 cm. through the center of the suture. The bowel wall is inverted as each of the two purse-string sutures is tightened about the catheter, and the loop of jejunum is fixed to the parietal peritoneum at the site of a stab wound by interrupted silk sutures. The catheter is also fixed by a silk suture placed in the skin.

An alternative method is that of Witzel. A purse-string suture is placed in the antimesenteric border of the jejunum. The catheter is inserted through a stab wound in the center of the circle, the purse-string suture tightened, and 3 to 4 cm. of proximal catheter is buried in the wall of the jejunum by three or four interrupted silk sutures placed over the catheter. This forms a tunnel and facilitates spontaneous closure of the enterostomy opening when the catheter is withdrawn. Spontaneous closure can also be aided by bringing the catheter through the omentum.

FEEDINGS

Many formulas have been developed for jejunostomy feedings. The main difficulty that arises is that hypertonic solutions introduced into the jejunum may cause cramps, diarrhea, and symptoms of the dumping syndrome. This is due to the rapid entrance of fluid into the lumen of the bowel from the blood in an attempt to make the contents of the jejunum isotonic, a function ordinarily assumed by the stomach. If these symptoms are prolonged, dehydration, hypernatremia, hyperchloremia, and azotemia may follow. This sequence of events can usually be prevented by making the jejunostomy feeding as isosmotic as possible and by introducing it slowly. An excellent method of giving the nutrient material in a slow but steady manner is by use of the Barron pump.[1] A formula suitable for use with this pump is shown in Table 12–5.

ILEOSTOMY

The great majority of patients with ulcerative colitis who need surgery will require a complete removal of the colon and rectum and an ileostomy. The greatest single factor in restoring these people to normal social and economic activity has been the development of the modern ileostomy appliance. No ileostomy appliance, however, will prevent leakage of bowel content with subsequent skin irritation, odor, and soiling of clothes unless the ileostomy itself has been well constructed. Thus, to a very large extent, the rehabilitation of these patients depends on a careful technique in the construction of their ileostomy. Just a few years ago many of them developed skin irritation, fistulas, prolapse, retraction, and intermittent small bowel obstruction. Today, almost all these complications can be avoided at the time the ileostomy is established.

POSITION

The site for the ileostomy on the abdominal wall is selected with care. Ordinarily the right lower quadrant is used. The ileostomy is placed where the disk of the appliance can be securely cemented to the skin. If the right lower quadrant is irregular due to the scars of a previous operation, the left lower quadrant or the right upper quadrant may be used. One selects the most convex point in this region, taking care that the edge of the ileostomy disk will not override the umbilicus, the anterior-superior spine, or the pubic hairline. If it does, they will interfere with the adherence of the appliance to the skin. A long, left paramedian incision is used for the colectomy so that the only incision in the right lower quadrant is the excision of a button of skin for the ileostomy. If the patient has a tendency to keloid formation, a linear incision at this site could interfere with proper adherence of the appliance. Moreover, these patients are likely to be malnourished and underweight. As they regain their weight, a depression at the site of a linear incision in the right lower quadrant would interfere with proper fixation of the ileostomy ring. Either a similar button of fascia is removed from the anterior and posterior rectus sheaths or these structures may be incised in a cruciate manner. The opening in the abdominal wall should fit the ileum snugly but not tightly.

FIXATION

Prolapse and retraction, formerly common complications of an ileostomy, have been eliminated by fixation of the mesentery of the terminal small bowel to the parietal peritoneum. This can be done by placing interrupted sutures uniting the mesentery to the undersurface of the abdominal wall up to the margin of the bowel. The blood vessels in the mesentery are carefully avoided. Sutures are not taken in the bowel wall to avoid the risk of a fistula.

Additional fixation is obtained by suture of the cut edge of the more proximal mesentery to the lateral and anterior abdominal wall, thus closing the right lumbar gutter. This also has the effect of preventing a 180-degree twist of the terminal ileum or herniation of more proximal small bowel.

STOMA

At one time bouts of temporary obstruction at the stoma were frequent in patients who had had an ileostomy established. This required frequent digital dilatations for the cramplike pain due to partial intestinal obstruction. Some years ago, Brooke,[2, 3] and later Turnbull,[4] pointed out that this was largely due to the induration and thickening of the protruding bowel as it became soiled by its own content. This has been almost entirely overcome by protecting the serosal surface of the protruding ileum by turning the bowel back upon itself. At first, this was done by excising the serosa from the distal 3 to 4 cm. of ileum and everting the muscularis and mucosa over the proximal protruding bowel. The edge of the mucosa was then sutured to the skin. The disadvantage of this was that it was difficult to avoid buttonholing the fragile mucosa and muscularis. The same protection to the serosa can be obtained by simply everting the entire thickness of the bowel and suturing the mucosa to the skin. If 2 inches of ileum is exteriorized, after eversion the ileostomy will protrude above the level of the skin about 1 inch. This is sufficient for good emptying into the ileostomy appliance without excessive protrusion. The cut margin of the bowel is sutured to the skin with interrupted fine catgut sutures around the entire circumference of the ileostomy stoma. Less reaction around the catgut will occur if the sutures are placed in the subcuticular layer of the skin.

APPLIANCE

A temporary ileostomy appliance is cemented to the skin over the ileostomy. A free space of $\frac{1}{8}$ to $\frac{3}{16}$ of an inch should be allowed between the edge of the bowel and the edge of the appliance to avoid pressure by the appliance on the bowel. Fixation of the adhesive is aided by first painting the surrounding skin with tincture of benzoin compound. The patient is measured for a permanent appliance before leaving the hospital. We prefer either the Torbot or the Perma-type permanent appliance. These can be obtained with varying degrees of convexity of the disk. The ileostomy kit contains not only the appliance, but also belts, cement, solvent, and instructions.

Before the patient is discharged from the hospital he or she should be carefully instructed in the care of the ileostomy. Two of the most important instructions are: (1) If the ileostomy appliance is loosened from the skin and leakage occurs, it must be recemented promptly. Skin irritation is very difficult to correct once it develops. It can, however, be prevented by never allowing the ileostomy content to soil the skin for longer than a few hours. (2) If there is swelling of the ileostomy so that the rigid edge of the ring presses on the side of the ileostomy, the appliance should be removed at once and replaced by another with a larger aperture. If one is not immediately available, a temporary appliance can be used. Persistent pressure on the side of the ileostomy may lead to a fistula at the skin level. All ileostomy content will then come from the fistulous opening rather than from the normal opening of the ileostomy, and the appliance will no longer adhere to the skin. In most instances a new ileostomy must then be constructed. Patients are advised to change their ileostomy appliance daily although some prefer to do it only once or twice a week. This is permissible as long as there is no sign of skin irritation. Patients quickly learn that keeping the appliance and skin meticulously clean is an important factor in eliminating odor.

COMPLICATIONS

All patients are instructed to contact their surgeon promptly if any complications occur such as skin irritation, obstruction, prolapse, or retraction. Temporary distal small bowel obstruction can usually be relieved by catheter irrigation of the ileostomy. If this is not successful, the small bowel should be decompressed from above by a long tube. If treated promptly, few patients will require laparotomy for relief of the obstruction.

REFERENCES

1. Barron, J.: Tube feeding of postoperative patients. S. Clin. North America *39:*1481–1491 (Dec.) 1959.
2. Brooke, B. N.: Management of ileostomy including its complications. Lancet *2:*102–104 (July 19) 1952.
3. Brooke, B. N.: Management of patient with colostomy or ileostomy. Postgrad. M. J. *30:*237–241 (May) 1954.
4. Turnbull, R. B., Jr.: Colectomy with simultaneous ileostomy as the surgical treatment of diffuse ulcerative colitis. Surgery *41:*843–856 (May) 1957.

Chapter Fourteen

VASCULAR MALFORMATIONS AND TUMORS

Vascular malformations and tumors comprise a group of lesions which is not homogeneous but has a probable common derivation. The study of these lesions poses certain difficulties because of their rarity, the difficulty of their recognition, and the uncertainty in some instances whether the lesion is a malformation or a true neoplasm. Relevant material can be found in Chapter Four on small bowel tumors, but a more complete discussion will appear here.

A classification of these malformations and tumors based on histopathologic features has been suggested by Gentry et al. (Table 14–1).[4] Each of these lesions (except multiple, noncontiguous, cavernous hemangiomas) has been reported to occur in the small intestine and in other parts of the gastrointestinal tract. In reviewing this subject, Gentry et al.[4] culled only 106 surgical and autopsy cases from 1,400,000 case records at the Mayo Clinic for an incidence of 0.008 percent.

TELANGIECTASIS

Telangiectasis refers to dilatation of existing blood vessels, whereas angiomas are made up of outgrowths of ectopic, endothelial-lined, blood-containing spaces. A hereditary type of telangiectasia was described by Osler[11] in 1901, although Rendu[13] was the first to associate familial epistaxis and multiple telangiectasia of the mucous membranes. For the diagnosis of hereditary telangiectasia to be made, the patient must have: (1) a history

Table 14–1. Vascular Malformations and Tumors of Small Intestine*

	TOTAL CASES IN LITERATURE 1839–1945	MAYO CLINIC SERIES TO JULY 1945
I. Benign vascular lesions		
A. Telangiectasis (hereditary and nonhereditary)	12†	0
B. Hemangioma		
1. Capillary hemangioma (simplex, mostly single)	2	0
2. Mixed capillary and cavernous hemangioma	5	5
3. Cavernous hemangioma		
a. Multiple phlebectasis (small cavernous)	53	53
b. Single polypoid (single cavernous)	0	10
c. Diffuse expansive (single contiguous)	15	2
d. Diffuse expansive (multiple noncontiguous)	0	0
II. Malignant vascular lesions		
A. Hemangioendothelioma	1	3
B. "Benign metastasizing hemangioma"	4	0
C. Kaposi's sarcoma	11	0
D. Angiosarcoma	1	0

* Adapted from Gentry et al.: Internat. Abstr. Surg. *88*:282, 288–304, 1949.
† Described as involving the gastrointestinal tract.

of repeated hemorrhages; (2) suitable lesions of the mucous membranes of the nasal or oral cavities, viscera, or skin; and (3) a familial occurrence. Characteristically, there is recurrent epistaxis in childhood or early adult life.[14] Angiomatous lesions appear on the skin or mucous membranes in early or middle adult life. Sublingual involvement is said to be common. On the other hand, the visceral manifestations may predominante without external stigmata. Gastrointestinal hemorrhage usually does not become evident until after the fourth decade. Occasionally, there are associated pulmonary arteriovenous fistulas.[10] To 1931, approximately 100 families were recorded.[5] Gentry et al.[4] found only 28 cases of visceral telangiectasia in the literature.

There is a second syndrome of rarer occurrence involving hemangiectatic hypertrophy of limbs (Parkes-Weber-Klippel syndrome), and in a case reported by Shepherd,[14] visceral (peritoneum, small bowel, and colon) nodular telangiectasia. This condition is not hereditary.

The treatment of gastrointestinal hemorrhage from these lesions is not satisfactory as their visceral involvement is too extensive. However, Vetto[16] has reported 11 patients with multiple, nonhereditary, diffuse telangiectasia of the small intestine in four of whom massive resection was carried out with apparent arrest of bleeding. He also pointed out a diagnostic procedure useful at laparotomy in which the submucosally located telangiectasia is demonstrable by pressing a glass slide against the side wall of the bowel. In cases with visceral involvement there is a tendency to spontaneous regression, but ultimately symptoms of bleeding return. The use of parenteral rutin[8] or moccasin venom[3] has been reported, but the efficacy of these treatments has not been confirmed.

HEMANGIOMAS

Other benign vascular lesions are classified as hemangiomas and are of three varieties: capillary hemangiomas, cavernous hemangiomas, or mixed types. Hemangiomas probably have their origin in embryonic sequestrations of mesodermal tissue. They may undergo acceleration of growth and become locally destructive or are lethal because of hemorrhage, obstruction, or perforation and sepsis.

Capillary hemangiomas may occur as single encapsulated tumors and consist of closely packed blood vessels with well-differentiated endothelium. They may appear as plaques or as pedunculated tumors which may cause intussusception and obstruction. Ulceration of their mucosal surface leads to hemorrhage and melena. Resection has been possible in the majority of reported cases.[4]

Cavernous hemangiomas consist of blood-filled spaces or sinuses lined by single or multiple layers of endothelial cells. Degenerative or sclerosing changes may be present as evidenced by hyalinization, edema, overgrowth of fibrous tissue, and calcification. The calcification may be observed on the plain film of the abdomen.[9] There are four kinds of cavernous hemangiomas. The first, the multiple phlebectasis type, is characterized by a multiplicity of small discrete lesions, which may be scattered throughout the gastrointestinal tract. The single polypoid type of cavernous hemangioma is often associated with ulceration, hemorrhage, and intestinal obstruction. Eighty percent of Gentry's lesions developed these complications.[4] The diffuse expansive cavernous hemangiomas are either single or multiple in their occurrence. Many involve 20 to 30 cm. of the gastrointestinal tract. A high proportion of these lesions are symptomatic, and the mortality from them is appreciable.

There is another group of hemangiomas that histologically and grossly shows features resembling both capillary and cavernous types. In common with all hemangiomas they ulcerate, bleed, obstruct, and perforate.

MALIGNANT VASCULAR TUMORS

The malignant counterparts of the benign vascular tumors are rarely encountered. Of the four such tumors listed in Table 14–1, there is much confusion surrounding the differentiation of hemangioendotheliomas from "benign metastasizing hemangiomas." Hemangioendotheliomas are made up of vascular tubes that have endothelial cells in their basic stroma and that demonstrate aggressive growth characteristics. They are usually situated in the submucosa and are lobulated. On palpation they suggest alternating firm and soft areas and sometimes show areas of degeneration. Because of a tendency to local lymph node metastasis, segmental resection including a generous area of mesenteric nodes is indicated.

Benign metastasizing hemangiomas are similar histologically, but are characterized by extensive metastases despite a seemingly benign histologic appearance. There is some question whether or not the metastases are separate tumors, and in fact the existence of this group as an entity is in doubt.

Kaposi's sarcoma, a malignant tumor of blood vascular elements and cavernous, blood-filled spaces, has a tendency to develop first on the extremities, but often progresses to involve the small intestine. It differs from hemangioendothelioma in this regard and also because there seems to be a male sex-linked feature. The course of the disease is invariably fatal.

Angiosarcoma is another type of malignant blood vessel tumor which has been reported to occur in the small intestine.[4] These tumors are composed of cells of the connective tissue type. Their course is generally fatal.

LOCALIZATION OF SITE OF BLEEDING

As mentioned previously, therapy of these lesions may be indicated by obstruction or perforation of the lesion. However, bleeding (melena) is the most common complication. The preoperative diagnosis of bleeding from lesions of the small intestine (1.4 percent of gastrointestinal hemorrhage) and especially from small bowel telangiectasia or angiomas can be most difficult.[15] The use of a long intestinal tube to obtain samples from various levels of the small intestine has merit in the actively bleeding cases.[1] Blood found in the aspirate at a certain level can be identified by the usual guaiac method or by radioactivity measurements if the patient is given tagged cells.[7, 12] Blood can also be identified on a suitably placed string by a Wood's lamp after fluorescein has been given parenterally.[6]

If, at surgery, no lesion is seen by external examination, Ferguson[2] has recommended aspirating the bowel at various levels. If blood is found, he suggests that the bowel should be opened and inspected proximally and distally. If no lesions are seen, a resection of 2 feet of bowel including the enterostomy site should be done. He has found this method to be effective and reported seven cases handled successfully. This procedure is of use only in actively bleeding cases.

REFERENCES

1. Brief, D. K., and Botsford, T. W.: Primary bleeding from the small intestine in adults. The surgical management. J.A.M.A. *184:*18–22 (Apr. 6) 1963.
2. Ferguson, L. K.: The diagnosis and management of bleeding from the lower intestine. Surgery *45:*352–354 (Feb.) 1959.
3. Figi, F. A., and Watkins, C. H.: Hereditary hemorrhagic telangiectasia. Ann. Otol. Rhin. & Laryng. *52:*330–341 (June) 1943.
4. Gentry, R. W., Dockerty, M. B., and Clagett, O. T.: Collective review; vascular malformations and vascular tumors of gastrointestinal tract. Internat. Abstr. Surg. *88:*281–323, 1949; *in* Surg. Gynec. & Obst. (Apr.) 1949.
5. Goldstein, H. I.: I. Goldstein's heredofamilial angiomatosis with recurring familial hemorrhages (Rendu-Osler-Weber's disease). Arch. Int. Med. *48:*836–865 (Nov.) 1931.
6. Haynes, W. F., Jr., Pittman, F. E., and Christakis, G.: Location of site of upper gastrointestinal tract hemorrhage by the fluorescein string test. Surgery *48:*821–827 (Nov.) 1960.
7. Healey, W. V., Riggins, R. C., White, R. L., et al.: An experimental method for localizing the source of intestinal bleeding. Surg. Gynec. & Obst. *112:*285–288 (Mar.) 1961.
8. Kushlan, S. D.: Gastro-intestinal bleeding in hereditary hemorrhagic telangiectasia; historical review and case report with gastroscopic findings and rutin therapy. Gastroenterology *7:*199–212 (Aug.) 1946.
9. Madell, S. H.: A case of hemangioma (angiomatosis) of the small intestine and mesentery; a radiographic clue to diagnosis. Radiology *69:*564–566 (Oct.) 1957.
10. Monroe, L. S., and Spencer, F. M.: The clinical significance of hereditary hemorrhagic telangiectasia. Gastroenterology *38:*906–911 (June) 1960.
11. Osler, W.: On a family form of recurring epistaxis, associated with multiple telangiectases of the skin and mucous membranes. Bull. Johns Hopkins Hosp. *12:*333–337 (Nov.) 1901.
12. Pillow, R. P., Hill, L. D., Ragen, P. A., et al.: Newer methods for localization of obscure small-bowel bleeding. J.A.M.A. *179:*23–26 (Jan. 6) 1962.
13. Rendu, M.: Épistaxis répétées chez un sujet porteur de petits angiomes cutanés et muqueux. Bull. et mém. Soc. med. d. hôp. de Paris *13:*731–733 (Oct. 23) 1896.
14. Shepherd, J. A.: Angiomatous conditions of gastrointestinal tract. Brit. J. Surg. *40:*409–421 (Mar.) 1953.
15. Thompson, H. L., and McGuffin, D. W.: Melena: study of underlying causes. J.A.M.A. *141:*1208–1213 (Dec. 24) 1949.
16. Vetto, R. M.: The management of multiple, diffuse telangiectasia of the small intestine. Surg. Gynec. & Obst. *115:*56–60 (July) 1962.

Chapter Fifteen

MESENTERIC VASCULAR INSUFFICIENCY

Ischemia and infarction of all or segments of the small intestine due to vascular disease[16, 22] have been recognized since Tiedemann[43] reported the first case of superior mesenteric artery occlusion in 1843. During the first hundred years since this report the only treatment was resection of the involved intestine, a procedure that frequently resulted in severe disturbances due to the short bowel syndrome if the patient was fortunate enough to survive the initial catastrophe. With the development of vascular surgery in the last 25 years it was inevitable that these techniques be applied to disease of the superior mesenteric artery. Since it is now feasible to deal directly with the two major causes of mesenteric artery occlusion (embolus and arteriosclerosis) many reports have appeared defining the problem, outlining the diagnostic features of small bowel ischemia, and reporting the results of a variety of treatment techniques. Progress has been slow only in the field of diagnosis. Table 15–1 classifies the various clinical syndromes of mesenteric vessel insufficiency.

ETIOLOGY AND DIAGNOSIS

Complete Occlusion of Superior Mesenteric Artery

Etiology

Jackson[16] has reviewed the literature prior to 1963 and has shown that 42 percent of acute arterial occlusions are due to emboli. Thirty-eight percent are due to gradual narrowing by obliterative arteriosclerosis with or

Table 15-1. Classification of Small Intestinal Ischemia Due to Vascular Disease

I. Superior mesenteric artery insufficiency
A. Acute occlusion
Embolism
Thrombosis
B. Intestinal angina
II. Nonocclusive infarction
III. Superior mesenteric vein occlusion

without superimposed acute thrombotic occlusion. In 20 percent of cases no obstructing lesion is found in the mesenteric vessels.[15] Rarely, physical manipulation of the aorta or superior mesenteric artery by surgical procedures[19] or arteriography[45] may be followed by mesenteric occlusion due to vasospasm, hematoma formation, or dislodgment of plaques. Penetrating abdominal wounds[28] and blunt abdominal trauma[29] have also resulted in damage to the superior mesenteric artery or vein with subsequent obstruction.

Diagnosis

Table 15-2 outlines the symptoms and signs of acute mesenteric occlusion as compiled by Jackson.[16] Abdominal pain that is steady, severe, and generalized is the most common symptom in acute occlusion. It may seem to be out of proportion to the physical findings since abdominal rigidity frequently is absent. The patient may be restless and apprehensive. After 12 hours, the temperature may rise and leukocytosis become evident. Shock may be apparent relatively early following the onset of occlusion, but its appearance after 12 or 24 hours is a sign of massive, irreversible necrosis. Distention on physical or radiographic examination is usually a late sign following occlusion.

The presence of auricular fibrillation or the history of a recent coronary occlusion is of great help in the diagnosis of embolism, but occasionally a silent coronary occlusion manifests itself for the first time by embolism to the superior mesenteric artery.[23]

Table 15-2. Clinical Manifestations of Acute Mesenteric Arterial Occlusion*

	PERCENT		PERCENT
Pain	100	Distention	80
Severe	65	Shock	60
Moderate	35	Rigidity	12
Leukocytosis	100		

* Adapted from Jackson, B. B.: Occlusion of the Superior Mesenteric Artery. Springfield, Charles C Thomas, 1963, p. 48.

There has been recent interest in various physiologic changes following superior mesenteric artery occlusion. In a study in dogs an increased small bowel motility, a decrease in the pH of the intestinal content, and a large loss of body potassium into the intestinal lumen were noted.[37] Marston[25] found a high rate (5 percent per hour) of blood volume contraction which he thought represented mainly plasma loss. The suggestion has been made that the recognition of these disturbances might be helpful in the diagnosis of mesenteric vascular occlusion.[37]

Following revascularization, hemorrhage with further loss of circulating volume,[26] loss of serum proteins,[46] continued loss of potassium, and liberation of a toxic substance into the circulation have been noted.[27]

Embolism

The superior mesenteric artery is particularly prone to obstruction by embolism because of its anatomic configuration parallel to the abdominal aorta, its large size, and its high flow rate. The embolus usually comes from a diseased valve or the atrium of the left heart or from a mural thrombus following cardiac infarction. The site of lodgment of the embolus is usually at an arteriosclerotic narrowing in the proximal artery or at the site of a major branching (usually at the mid-colic branch) where the lumen of the main channel suddenly narrows. Following the embolism, a secondary thrombus which may propagate distally or proximally usually forms. Another major sequela is the development of vasospasm in the distal artery. The bowel initially shows a blanched appearance due to the vasospasm and attendant loss of blood. Owing to anoxia, contractility of the bowel is lost, and large blue areas appear. After four to six hours of occlusion the entire bowel wall becomes cyanotic and blood-soaked because of an increase in permeability of blood vessel walls.[10]

Thrombosis

Thrombosis of the superior mesenteric artery is superimposed on arteriosclerotic narrowing of this vessel. The symptoms of this catastrophe are identical to embolic occlusion except that occasionally an antecedent history of intestinal angina can be elicited. Rarely thrombosis is superimposed on periarteritis nodosa involving smaller branches of the superior mesenteric artery, and in this instance, smaller areas of infarction are the rule.[6]

NONOCCLUSIVE INFARCTION

Infarction of the small intestine can occur without demonstrable occlusion of the superior mesenteric artery. The common denominator of all the possible associated conditions is a reduced blood flow to the small bowel.[8]

Thus, congestive failure,[14] diabetic coma, infection, hypovolemia, or even vasopressor therapy [13, 15] are capable of producing changes all the way from patchy necrosis of the antimesenteric border of the bowel to gangrene of the entire gastrointestinal tract.[24] As a rule infarction does not occur suddenly, but may develop slowly over a period of days or weeks. Even with extensive changes in the bowel wall, thrombosis is seldom found in the proximal superior mesenteric vessels, but some clotted blood may be seen in the vasa recta.

INTESTINAL ANGINA

The term "intestinal angina" is aptly descriptive of a syndrome of generalized abdominal pain, usually postprandial, caused by a relative deficiency of the blood supply to the small bowel in the digestive phase.[7] Marked weight loss occurs because of voluntary starvation in an effort to avoid symptoms and also because of malabsorption of fat and protein.[4, 5] Physical examination may be unrevealing except for evidence of severe malnutrition and the finding of a systolic bruit near the umbilicus.

The lesion causing this condition is arteriosclerotic narrowing, varying in degree, of the superior mesenteric artery. Subjects with complete occlusion of the superior mesenteric artery without symptoms have been described,[39] and conversely, patients have had severe symptoms with only a minimal narrowing. The suggestion of Mikkelsen[31] and Morris et al.[34] has merit;

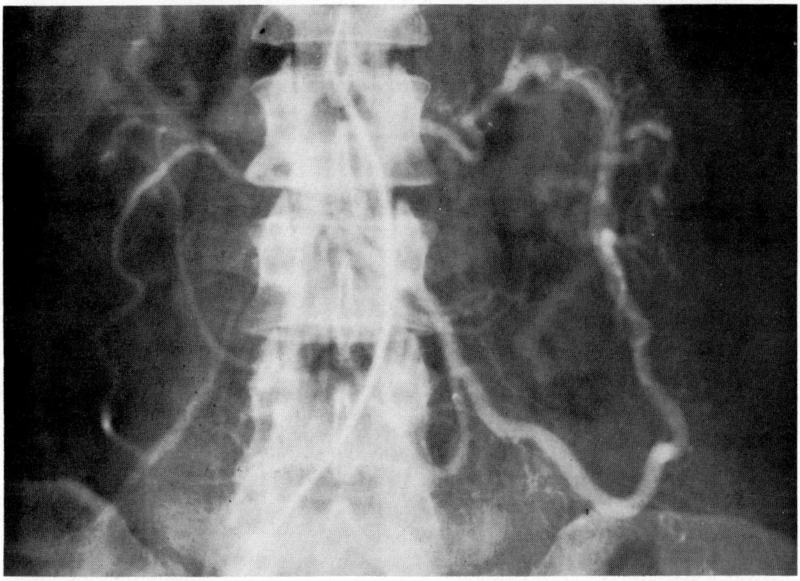

Figure 15–1. Retrograde femoral aortogram showing absence of superior mesenteric artery filling due to block at the origin of that artery. Note the collateral blood supply through the inferior mesenteric, the left colon arcuate, and the middle colic arteries.

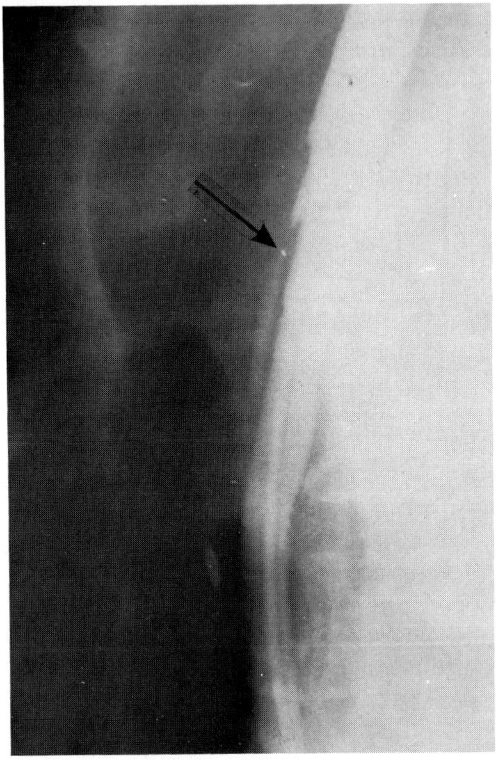

Figure 15–2. Lateral view of superior mesenteric artery obstruction.

that two of the three arteries (celiac, superior mesenteric, and inferior mesenteric) supplying the abdominal gastrointestinal tract must be involved with occlusive disease before the condition becomes clinically evident.

The diagnosis can only be made by aortography either by retrograde brachial injection or retrograde femoral catheterization (Fig. 15–1). Lateral views of the superior mesenteric and celiac artery takeoffs are essential (Fig. 15–2).

The exact incidence of this syndrome is unknown because of the hazards of aortography and because, even with demonstrable narrowing of the superior mesenteric artery, abdominal pain may be unrelated to vascular insufficiency. This syndrome is most common in the middle-aged male with disabling arteriosclerotic disease in the cerebral, femoral, or coronary arteries. A large proportion of these patients progress to acute occlusion.

SUPERIOR MESENTERIC VENOUS OBSTRUCTION

Infarction of the small intestine due to occlusion of the superior mesenteric vein has been estimated to occur in from 15 to 45 percent of all significant mesenteric vascular accidents.[9, 17, 30, 36, 44] In many cases the

Table 15-3. Disorders Predisposing to Mesenteric Vein Thrombosis

Hypercoagulable states
Carcinomatosis
Polycythemia
Local venous congestion and stasis
Hepatic cirrhosis
Extrinsic pressure on portal system
Direct injury to mesenteric veins
Trauma
Pyelophlebitis secondary to intraperitoneal suppuration
Radiation

venous thrombosis is associated with a variety of other clinical disorders as outlined in Table 15-3. These include hypercoagulable states, local stasis in the mesenteric vein, and injury to the superior mesenteric vein. In a significant proportion of cases (25 to 55 percent) no known predisposing cause can be demonstrated.[2, 17] It has been pointed out that many of these patients have previous or associated peripheral idiopathic thrombophlebitis.[35, 38]

The clinical manifestations of superior mesenteric venous thrombosis are different from acute arterial obstruction in that the course is less devastating.[35] Frequently mild symptoms such as anorexia and ill-defined abdominal discomfort associated with changes in bowel habits occur for days or weeks before the onset of severe symptoms. Following these initial symptoms, abdominal pain with vomiting may occur and increase in severity.

On examination low-grade fever is frequently the only finding. The abdomen does not often show spasm or rebound tenderness. In this respect there is a marked similarity to arterial occlusion. Other findings include a leukocytosis and the presence of serosanguineous fluid in the peritoneal cavity.

Examination of the involved intestine shows it to be markedly thickened, edematous, and cyanotic, with the lumen filled with dark bloody fluid.[35] The veins on cut section extrude thrombi, and the arteries show pulsation.

TREATMENT OF MESENTERIC VASCULAR INSUFFICIENCY

Distribution of Occlusions or Stenoses

Kümmell[21] has reported a postmortem study of 42 subjects over 40 years of age taken at random in which 17 showed severe stenotic changes in the proximal portion of the superior mesenteric artery. Peripheral branches were rarely involved. Derrick et al.[7] confirmed this finding. Another study revealed that the narrowest point of the superior mesenteric artery in 75 autopsied patients was 0.25 to 1 cm. distal to the aortic orifice.[1]

The distribution of occlusions has been studied by Johnson and Baggenstoss.[18] The autopsy files of the Mayo Clinic, covering examinations between

1911 and November 1945, yielded 60 cases of mesenteric arterial occlusion and 12 cases of mesenteric artery and vein occlusion. Fifty-seven of the 60 involved only the superior mesenteric artery. Of these 57, 22 involved only the proximal artery and 18 involved the proximal artery and peripheral branches. Twenty-three cases had an infarction which, if resected, was extensive enough to preclude life.

In another autopsy study, Glotzer and Shaw[12] reviewed 31 cases of small bowel infarction at the Massachusetts General Hospital. Of these 31 cases, 22 were due to occlusion of the superior mesenteric artery and in 9 there was infarction without occlusion. Of the 22 occlusions, in 50 percent it would have been feasible to treat the patient successfully by arterial surgery and 79 percent could have been treated successfully by a combination of arterial surgery and resection.

It would seem from these autopsy studies that the majority of the acute and chronic occlusions of the superior mesenteric artery, if treated early, are amenable to direct surgical attack on the artery.

REVIEW OF CASES

The first report of direct surgical intervention on the superior mesenteric artery was submitted by Klass[20] in 1951. Although his first two patients succumbed in the postoperative period following embolectomy, the feasibility of the procedure was established, especially since the distal mesenteric vessels were found to be patent. The first successful embolectomy was performed also in 1951 but not reported until 1960 by Stewart et al.[42] The year 1951, therefore, marks the dividing line between the purely resective phase of treatment, first reported to be successful by Elliot[11] in 1895, and the restoration of blood flow or resective treatment or both of recent times. The world's literature concerning embolectomy up to 1964 has been summarized by Laufman et al., who found only 10 successful cases with or without supplemental resection of infarcted bowel.[22]

The surgical treatment of acute thrombosis has likewise been reviewed by Laufman et al.,[22] who found 12 successful thromboendarterectomies or other reconstructive procedures in the literature, including the first thromboendarterectomy reported in 1958.[40]

Intestinal angina was first managed successfully by Shaw and Maynard[40] in 1957 by endarterectomy (reported in 1958). The largest series of such patients has been reported by Morris et al.[33] who treated 12 cases of celiac and mesenteric occlusive disease, largely by bypass operations. The successful case of Starzl and Trippel[41] deserves note since an endarterectomy was done on the renal, superior mesenteric, and aortoceliac arteries in one stage for hypertension, intestinal angina, and intermittent claudication. It should be noted that there are no long-term follow-up studies on patients with intestinal angina or acute infarction who were treated surgically.

Surgical Management

Diagnosis at Laparotomy

The differentiation of acute arterial occlusion from venous occlusion can be made from the gross findings at laparotomy. If there is marked thickening, edema, and cyanosis of all or part of the small intestine, and if the arteries pulsate normally, the diagnosis of mesenteric venous obstruction can be made with reasonable security. If there are signs of infarction (a blanched appearance early and a blood-soaked, deep blue appearance late) with absence of pulsations of the artery and its branches, arterial occlusion is probable. Ordinarily with embolism, the embolus can be palpated at about the mid-colic branch takeoff, and there are palpable pulsations proximally and a collapsed vessel distally. At times, arteriotomy is necessary to make the differentiation between embolus and thrombosis. With far-advanced gangrenous changes in the small intestine, the differentiation is academic and only a resection of involved intestine is indicated.

Embolism and Thrombosis

Ordinarily the approach to the superior mesenteric artery is from below the transverse mesocolon. With downward traction on the small bowel mesentery and upward traction on the transverse mesocolon, the superior mesenteric artery stands out as a taut cord. The inferior leaf of the mesocolon is incised and the inferior border of the pancreas dissected so as to retract the pancreas superiorly (Fig. 1–7). After isolation of the artery and the application of proximal and distal clamps, the embolus, if present, can be extracted through an appropriately placed arteriotomy. If a palpable thickening proves to be an area of arteriosclerosis, endarterectomy can be accomplished.[3] With arteriosclerotic obstruction, a C-clamp placed proximally on the aorta allows the necessary intraluminal exposure to the superior mesenteric artery origin. Another approach through the gastrocolic omentum might be considered if the inframesocolic exposure is not feasible. At times the inframesocolic or transgastrocolic approach to the origin of the superior mesenteric artery is hazardous. In these instances, reflection of the left colon to the right with elevation of the spleen and pancreas will allow a retroperitoneal approach to this area. The use of heparin in the distal arterial tree is recommended before the occluding distal clamp is applied. After endarterectomy, the intima at the distal extent of the endarterectomy must be sutured to the vessel wall to prevent dissection. In closing the arteriotomy incision a patch graft is often used. After blood flow is reestablished, the bowel must be carefully examined for irreversible necrosis necessitating resection. After massive resection, consideration should be given to reversing a short loop of terminal small bowel (see Chapter Six).

Postoperatively, systemic heparinization is not indicated. Reexploration in the postoperative period as carried out by Shaw and Maynard[40] should be considered, especially if any bowel of questionable viability was left in the abdomen. Most patients require large amounts of plasma or blood in the immediate postoperative period.

Alternate procedures of bypass graft, as advocated by Morris et al.,[33] or division of the superior mesenteric artery just below the duodenum with reanastomosis to the aorta, as advocated by Miller and DiMare,[32] should be considered if the direct approach to the proximal superior mesenteric artery is not feasible.

Intestinal Angina

In the surgical management of intestinal angina, three procedures have been successful. As mentioned previously, these include thromboendarterectomy as used by Shaw and Maynard[40] in their first successfully treated case, reimplantation of the superior mesenteric artery into the aorta,[32] or aortic bypass graft as advocated by Morris et al.[33] in the largest available series. Morris points out that difficulties in control of the proximal vessel are avoided by his procedure.

Mesenteric Vein Occlusion

The treatment of mesenteric vein occlusion is primarily resective. The surgeon should keep in mind that thromboses frequently extend into the veins beyond the grossly infarcted bowel. Therefore, the limits of resection should encompass all gross disease and a margin of normal tissue.[35] In the postoperative period anticoagulation seems warranted and should be continued for from 6 to 10 weeks.[35]

REFERENCES

1. Arkin, A.: A clinical and pathological study of periarteritis nodosa: A report of five cases, one histologically healed. Am. J. Path. *6:*401–426 (July) 1930.
2. Berry, F. B., and Bougas, J. A.: Agnogenic venous mesenteric thrombosis. Ann. Surg. *132:*450–474 (Sept.) 1950.
3. Brittain, R. S., and Earley, T. K.: Emergency thrombo-endarterectomy of the superior mesenteric artery: report of four cases. Ann. Surg. *158:*138–143 (July) 1963.
4. Dardik, H., Seidenberg, B., Parker, J. G., et al.: Intestinal angina with malabsorption treated by elective revascularization. Case report and review of the literature with emphasis on absorption studies. J.A.M.A. *194:*1206–1210 (Dec. 13) 1965.
5. DeLangen, C. D.: Steatorrhoea and intestinal circulation. Acta. med. scandinav. *146:*7–19, 1953.
6. DeMuth, W. E., Jr., Fitts, W. T., Jr., and Patterson, L. T.: Mesenteric vascular occlusion. Internat. Abstr. Surg. *108:*209–223 (Mar.) 1959; *in* Surg. Gynec. & Obst. *108* (Mar.) 1959.
7. Derrick, J. R., Pollard, H. S., and Moore, R. M.: The pattern of arteriosclerotic narrowing of the celiac and superior mesenteric arteries. Ann. Surg. *149:*684–689 (May) 1959.

8. Drucker, W. R., Davis, J. H., Holden, W. D., et al.: Hemorrhagic necrosis of the intestine. A clinical syndrome: presence without organic vascular occlusion. Arch. Surg. *89:*42–53 (July) 1964.
9. Duncan, R. D., Ferrell, T. E., and Hansbro, G. L.: Acute mesenteric venous thrombosis. Am. J. Surg. *83:*205–208 (Feb.) 1952.
10. Dunphy, J. E., and Zollinger, R.: Mesenteric vascular occlusion. New England J. Med. *211:*708–711 (Oct. 18) 1934.
11. Elliot, J. W.: The operative relief of gangrene of intestine due to occlusion of the mesenteric vessels. Ann. Surg. *21:*9–23 (Jan.) 1895.
12. Glotzer, D. J., and Shaw, R. S.: Massive bowel infarction; an autopsy study assessing the potentialities of reconstructive vascular surgery. New England J. Med. *260:*162–167 (Jan. 22) 1959.
13. Granata, L., Huvos, A., and Gregg, D. E.: Hemodynamic changes in coronary and mesenteric arterial beds following sympathetic nerve stimulation. Physiologist *4:*42, 1961.
14. Hamilton, M. D., Barnett, A. J., and Lowe, T. E.: Ischaemic episodes in cardiac failure: acute arterial insufficiency with and without structural blockage. M. J. Australia *2:*93–95 (July 16) 1955.
15. Hardy, J. D., and Alican, F.: Ischemic gangrene without major organic vascular occlusion: an enlarging concept. Surgery *50:*107–114 (July) 1961.
16. Jackson, B. B.: Occlusion of the Superior Mesenteric Artery. Springfield, Ill., Charles C Thomas, 1963.
17. Jenson, C. B., and Smith, G. A.: Clinical study of 51 cases of mesenteric infarction. Surgery *40:*930–937 (Nov.) 1956.
18. Johnson, C. C., and Baggenstoss, A. H.: Mesenteric vascular occlusion; study of 60 cases of occlusion of arteries, and of 12 cases of occlusion of both arteries and veins. Proc. Staff Meet. Mayo Clin. *24:*649–656 (Dec. 21) 1949.
19. Johnson, J. T.: Thrombosis and embolism following abdominal operations. Surg. Gynec. & Obst. *3:*110–115 (July) 1906.
20. Klass, A. A.: Embolectomy in acute mesenteric occlusion. Ann. Surg. *134:*913–917 (Nov.) 1951.
21. Kümmell, R.: Über die Sklerose der Eingeweidearterien der Bauchhöhle. Zentralbl. allg. Path. *17:*129–134 (Feb. 28) 1906.
22. Laufman, H., Nora, P. F., and Mittelpunkt, A. I.: Mesenteric blood vessels: advances in surgery and physiology. Arch. Surg. *88:*1021–1044 (June) 1964.
23. Laufman, H., and Scheinberg, S.: Arterial and venous mesenteric occlusion: Analysis of forty-four cases. Am. J. Surg. *58:*84–92 (Oct.) 1942.
24. Longo, O. F.: Infarto intestinomesenterico inexplicado o apoplejia intestinomesenterica. Prensa méd. argent. *34:*419–421 (Feb. 28) 1947.
25. Marston, A.: Causes of death in mesenteric arterial occlusion. I. Local and general effects of devascularization of the bowel. Ann. Surg. *158:*952–959 (Dec.) 1963.
26. Marston, A.: Causes of death in mesenteric arterial occlusion. II. Observations on revascularization of the ischemic bowel. Ann. Surg. *158:*960–970 (Dec.) 1963.
27. Mavor, G. E., Lyall, A. D., Chrystal, K. M., et al.: Mesenteric infarction as a vascular emergency. The clinical problems. Brit. J. Surg. *50:*219–225 (Sept.) 1962.
28. May, A. G., Lipchik, E. O., and DeWeese, J. A.: Repair of hepatic and superior mesenteric artery injury: Patency demonstrated by aortography. Ann. Surg. *162:*869–872 (Nov.) 1965.
29. McCune, W. S., Keshishian, J. M., and Blades, B.: Mesenteric thrombosis following blunt abdominal trauma. Ann. Surg. *135:*606–614 (May) 1952.
30. Mersheimer, W. L., Winfield, J. M., and Frankhauser, R. L.: Mesenteric vascular occlusion; report of 5 successful resections. Arch. Surg. *66:*752–768 (June) 1953.
31. Mikkelsen, W. P.: Intestinal angina: its surgical significance. Am. J. Surg. *94:*262–267 (Aug.) 1957.
32. Miller, H. I., and DiMare, S. A.: Mesenteric infarction; report of a case of superior-mesenteric-artery embolectomy and small-bowel resection, with recovery. New England J. Med. *259:*512–515 (Sept. 11) 1958.
33. Morris, G. C., Jr., Crawford, E. S., Cooley, D. A., at al.: Revascularization of celiac and superior mesenteric arteries. Arch. Surg. *84:*95–107 (Jan.) 1962.
34. Morris, G. C., Jr., and DeBakey, M. E.: Abdominal angina—diagnosis and surgical treatment. J.A.M.A. *176:*89–92 (Apr. 15) 1961.

35. Naitove, A., and Weismann, R. E.: Primary mesenteric venous thrombosis. Ann. Surg. *161:*516–523 (Apr.) 1965.
36. Nanson, E. M.: Vascular lesions producing the "acute abdomen." S. Clin. North America *40:*1241–1259 (Oct.) 1960.
37. Nelson, R. A.: Effect of reduced arterial pressure and flow on intestinal function. Surg. Gynec. & Obst. *120:*1221–1224 (June) 1965.
38. North, J. P., and Wollenman, O. J., Jr.: Venous mesenteric occlusion in course of migrating thrombophlebitis. Surg. Gynec. & Obst. *95:*665–671 (Dec.) 1952.
39. Rob, C. G., and Owen, K.: Ligation of both the coeliac axis and superior mesenteric artery with survival of the patient. Brit. J. Surg. *44:*247–249 (Nov.) 1956.
40. Shaw, R. S., and Maynard, E. P., III: Acute and chronic thrombosis of the mesenteric arteries associated with malabsorption; a report of two cases successfully treated by thromboendarterectomy. New England J. Med. *258:*874–878 (May 1) 1958.
41. Starzl, T. E., and Trippel, O. H.: Reno-mesentero-aorto-iliac thromboendarterectomy in patient with malignant hypertension. Surgery *46:*556–564 (Sept.) 1959.
42. Stewart, G. D., Sweetman, W. R., Westphal, K., et al.: Superior mesenteric artery embolectomy. Ann. Surg. *151:*274–278 (Feb.) 1960.
43. Tiedemann, F.: Von der Verengung und Schliessung der Pulsadern in Krankheiten. Heidelberg and Leipzig, K. Groos, 1843.
44. Uricchio, J. F., Calenda, D. G., and Freedman, D.: Mesenteric vascular occlusion; analysis of 13 cases with report of 2 cases with survival following extensive intestinal resection. Ann. Surg. *139:*206–217 (Feb.) 1954.
45. Wilder, R. J., and Steichen, F. M.: Necrosis of the entire gastrointestinal tract following translumbar aortography. Arch. Surg. *80:*198–203 (Feb.) 1960.
46. Zuidema, G. D., Turcotte, J. G., Wolfman, E. F., Jr., et al.: Metabolic studies in acute small-bowel ischemia. Arch. Surg. *85:*130–135 (July) 1962.

Chapter Sixteen

TRANSPLANTATION

AUTOTRANSPLANTATION AND HOMOTRANSPLANTATION

The small intestine has not escaped the attention of the surgeon-biologist who has found that transplantation problems of the small bowel are basically similar to those of other organs. Lillehei[22] was directed to small bowel transplantation in the course of work on shock. In 1959 he reported on a successful autografting procedure of the small intestine in dogs and showed that cooling the bowel to 5° C. prolonged the period of time that the intestine could be safely stored in vitro before autotransplantation.[24]

Homotransplantation of the entire small intestine results in rejection of the host by the graft with death of the animal, since at autopsy a normal graft is found.[2, 23] Homografting of smaller 10 to 20 cm. segments of the small intestine to either the neck or in continuity with the intestinal stream results in rejection of the graft in the usual time interval.

There are problems other than homograft survival involved in small bowel transplantation that involve the lymphatic and nervous pathways. Studies have demonstrated that after autologous transplantation, the lymphatics regenerate in two to three weeks.[1, 23] Ballinger et al.[1] have suggested that the complete denervation that follows autotransplantation in dogs causes weight loss, diarrhea, altered barium patterns, malabsorption of fat, and loss of villi. They found that after denervation of the intact small intestine, these functions did not return to normal until after a four- to six-month period.

In summary the mechanics of small bowel homografting have been solved, but as in other areas, clinical usage is delayed until the rejection mechanism can be controlled.

THE USE OF THE SMALL INTESTINE AS GRAFTS

The small intestine lends itself to a variety of uses as an adjunct or a substitute because of its accessibility, its presence in lengths beyond physio-

Table 16–1. Clinical Uses of Small Intestinal Grafts

SITE OF TRANSPLANT	FUNCTION	HUMAN APPLICATION
Patch to urinary bladder	Enlarge bladder capacity	Interstitial cystitis Tuberculous cystitis
Ureter	Replace resected segment of ureter	Trauma, tumors, strictures of ureter
Ureter to skin	Urinary conduit and pouch	Total cystectomy, vesicovaginal fistula, hydronephrosis, ectopic vesicae, cord bladder
Cervical, thoracic, and abdominal esophagus	Alimentary continuity	Carcinoma, lye stricture, esophagitis
Stomach	Reservoir	Small stomach syndrome
Stomach remnant to duodenum	Convert Billroth II resection to Billroth I	Dumping syndrome
Reversed loop between stomach remnant and duodenum or jejunum	Retard gastric emptying	Dumping syndrome

logic needs, its polarity of transport, and its distensibility. The small intestine can be used as a patch graft or a replacement for a hollow viscus, or it can be used as a tube to replace a deficit in the length of a duct or esophagus. It can be used as a free graft with subsequent revascularization or as a pedicle graft with an uninterrupted blood supply. A summary of clinical uses is found in Table 16–1.

UROLOGIC USES

Varieties

The urologic uses of the small intestine have been reviewed by Pyrah.[29] Mikulicz has been credited by Tasker[34] as performing the first ileocystoplasty in 1898. In patients with major losses of bladder capacity due to resection or destruction by disease, bladder wall replacement by a patch of ileum has proved satisfactory. Goodwin[10] recommends this procedure in the treatment of contracted bladders due to interstitial cystitis or tuberculosis.

According to Melnikoff,[25] Schoemaker in 1906 first used a loop of ileum to replace a segment of ureter. When deficiencies in ureteral length cannot be remedied by plastic procedures using other areas of the urinary tract, appropriately placed ileal loops can restore urinary continuity after resection of tumors, strictures, or fistulas, or after injuries to the ureter.[11, 26, 29]

Ileum has also proved useful as a urinary conduit to abdominal skin after resection of the urinary bladder,[3, 4] or for urinary diversion in the treatment of vesicovaginal fistula, bilateral hydronephrosis, spina bifida, spinal injury, or ectopia vesicae.[29] Its advantages, listed in Table 16–2, reflect the disadvantages associated with the use of the colon for urinary diversion.[7, 8, 9] The principal disadvantages are: (1) it is a time-consuming

Table 16-2. Advantages of "Ileal Loop" Procedure*

No fecal contamination
No stasis
No reabsorption
No restriction on radical pelvic surgery
No sphincter dependence
Adaptable for staging
Adaptable for most dilated ureters
Adaptable for subsequent pelvic irradiation
Permits sacrifice of lower portion of ureters
Single external stoma
Ease of retrograde studies
Freedom from catheters
No inherent tendency to infection

* From Dowd, J. B., and Shah, S.: S. Clin. North America *45:*742 (June) 1965.

procedure that must be carried out in a meticulous manner if complications are to be avoided and a good permanent result obtained; and (2) the patient must continue to wear a properly fitting external collection appliance. Although the ileal loop procedure has failed to reverse the sequelae of large, adynamic ureters, it probably represents the best method that we have for urinary diversion at the present time, except in the preterminal cancer patient. Here the disadvantages of ureterosigmoidostomy are less important since the long-term result is not a consideration.

In an effort to improve the usual segments of ileum used for conduction and storage, Shoemaker[33] removed all the ileal mucosa and formed a reversed seromuscular graft. This had inherent muscular tone with expulsive force, and the problem of electrolyte and nitrogenous waste resorption was eliminated. Modifications of this technique are still being developed, and its exact usefulness remains to be determined. Hirschhorn[16] has suggested the use of ileum as a sleeve to restore function to a diseased, dilated, and incompetent ureter. A length of ileum with its vascular pedicle was isolated, stripped of its mucosa, and applied as an isoperistaltic sleeve around the intact ureter. Early postoperative studies indicated absence of reflux and complete restoration of ureteral function and tone.

Technique of Construction of Ileal Loop

The important points in the construction of an ileal loop are illustrated in Figure 16–1. As for ulcerative colitis, the most convex portion of the right lower quadrant is chosen for the ileostomy stoma. A 2 to 3 cm. button of skin with anterior fascia is removed at that point. A left paramedian incision is then made, the sigmoid colon mobilized, and the left ureter identified. The left ureter is divided low in the pelvis and freed proximally; care must be taken to preserve the periureteral tissue that contains its blood supply. It is then brought through an opening in the base of the sigmoid mesentery

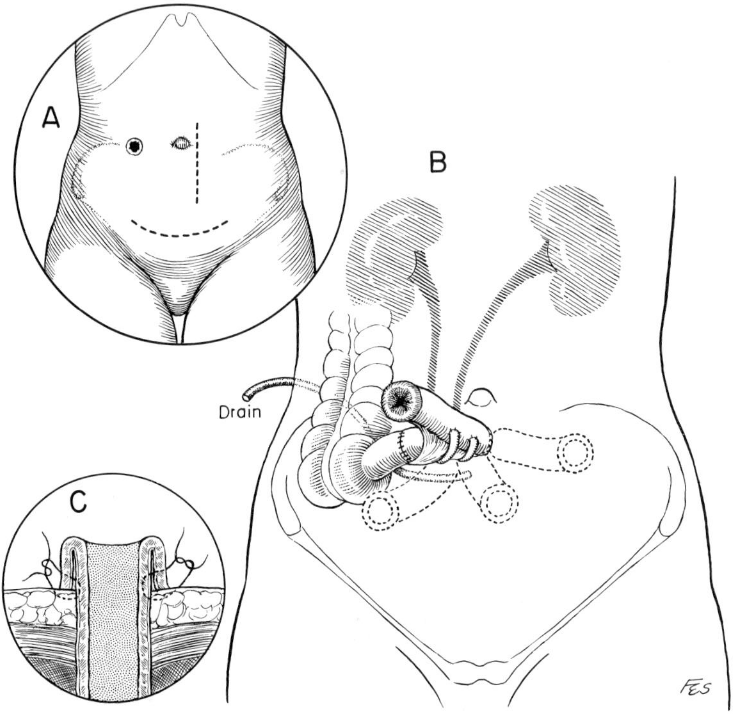

Figure 16–1. Technique of construction of ileal loop. *A,* Skin incisions and placement of stoma. *B,* Gastrointestinal and urinary reconstruction. *C,* Maturation of external stoma.

so that it will cross to the site of its anastomosis to the ileal loop without kinking. The right ureter is mobilized in a similar manner. A segment of terminal ileum, approximately 4 to 6 inches in length, is selected for the ileal loop. This segment is usually about 6 inches proximal to the ileocecal valve. If the terminal ileum has been injured by pelvic irradiation, a more proximal loop of ileum is chosen. The vascular pedicle to the isolated loop should contain at least two large pulsating vessels. It should be kept in mind that the ileal loop is designed to be a conduit and not a substitute bladder for urinary storage. If it is made too long, the risk of infarction, reabsorption, and infection are introduced. Small bowel continuity is reestablished by end-to-end anastomosis anterior to the isolated loop. The proximal end of the loop is closed. After the distal end of the loop is brought through the abdominal wall, avoiding distortion or constriction of the loop, each ureter is anastomosed to the loop near the closed end. A meticulous anastomosis is made with fine, interrupted, catgut sutures uniting the mucosa of the ileum to the spatulated ureter. An external row of fine, interrupted, silk sutures is then placed to protect this anastomosis, care being taken that the silk does not penetrate the lumen of the bowel or ureter.

The apertures created by the anastomosis of the left ureter to the ileal loop are then obliterated. The pelvis is drained either through the right flank or through the lower end of the incision. After closure of the laparotomy incision, the full thickness of the projecting ileum is then turned back on itself and sutured to the skin as is done for patients with ulcerative colitis.

Catheters are not placed in the ileum or ureters except under special circumstances. A temporary ileostomy appliance is cemented to the skin in the operating room at the conclusion of the operative procedure.

GASTROINTESTINAL TRACT USES

The use of jejunum in reconstruction of the esophagus after resection for esophagitis, lye stricture, or carcinoma has been recommended.[13, 18, 36] In those instances of lower esophageal replacement, the graft retains its superior mesenteric vessel pedicle. Carcinomas of the cervical esophagus present a special problem in treatment. A number of surgeons have used a free graft of a segment of jejunum, vascularized from cervical vessels, to bridge the gap in cervical esophagus after resection.[27, 30, 32]

The use of a jejunal pouch to improve or restore the reservoir function of the stomach after total[14] or subtotal[20, 21] gastrectomy has been investigated. Commonly, a triple-limbed jejunal pouch is constructed and interposed between the esophagus or gastric remnant and the small intestine. A good to excellent response has been reported as far as appetite, reservoir function, and fat and nitrogen absorption are concerned. Refractory anemias and severe dumping symptoms have been benefited. Unfortunately, clinical experience with this procedure is limited to only a few patients with short-term follow-up observations.

Jejunal isoperistaltic loops have been used after Billroth II gastrectomy to convert the gastrojejunostomy to a gastroduodenostomy. This procedure, known as Henley's remedial operation, has been reported to be effective in the surgical treatment of dumping.[15]

The polarity of flow through segments of small intestine has also been utilized in the treatment of the postgastrectomy dumping syndrome. Thus, a short segment of jejunum 2 to 3 inches long has been interposed in an antiperistaltic position between the gastric remnant and the jejunum in dogs and patients.[17, 28, 31] The patients so treated were said to have been benefited symptomatically and showed improvement in functional studies.

MISCELLANEOUS

Other uses of small intestinal grafts include procedures to replace lost anal sphincteric function,[35] to replace diseased colonic mucosa, to supplement a deficient coronary[19] or renal circulation, and to close diaphragmatic and peritoneal defects.[5, 6, 12, 19, 35]

REFERENCES

1. Ballinger, W. F., 2d, Christy, M. G., and Ashby, W. B.: Autotransplantation of the small intestine: the effect of denervation. Surgery *52:*151–164 (July) 1962.
2. Barnett, W. O., Truett, G., and Stone, J.: Experimental small-bowel homografts. Am. J. Digest. Dis. *7:*833–838 (Sept.) 1962.
3. Bricker, E. M.: Symposium on clinical surgery; bladder substitution after pelvic evisceration. S. Clin. North America *30:*1511–1521 (Oct.) 1950.
4. Bricker, E. M., Butcher, H. R., and McAfee, C. A.: Late results of bladder substitution with isolated ileal segments. Surg. Gynec. & Obst. *99:*469–482 (Oct.) 1954.
5. Brody, G. S., and McCorriston, J. R.: Experimental transplantation of small bowel mucosa to the rectum. Plast. & Reconstruct. Surg. *28:*12–25 (July) 1961.
6. Cockett, A. T., and Winters, C. C.: Revascularization of the ischemic kidney by means of an ileac loop. Am. J. Surg. *104:*543–550 (Oct.) 1962.
7. Dowd, J. B., and Shah, S.: Technique of uretero-ileal-cutaneous anastomosis ("the ileal loop"). S. Clin. North America *45:*741–750 (June) 1965.
8. Dowd, J. B., and Velasco, C.: Urologic uses of the small and large intestine. S. Clin. North America *44:*849–858 (June) 1964.
9. Flint, L. D., and Colcock, B. P.: Technique of ileal conduit for ureteral diversion. S. Clin. North America *40:*761–766 (June) 1960.
10. Goodwin, W. E., Turner, R. D., and Winter, C. C.: Results of ileocystoplasty. J. Urol. *80:*461–466 (Dec.) 1958.
11. Goodwin, W. E., Winter, C. C., and Turner, R. D.: Replacement of the ureter by small intestine: clinical application and results of the ileal ureter. J. Urol. *81:*406–418 (Mar.) 1959.
12. Hammer, J. M., Seay, P. H., Hill, E. J., et al.: Intestinal segments as internal pedicle grafts. Arch. Surg. *71:*625–642 (Oct.) 1955.
13. Harrison, A. W.: Transthoracic small bowel substitution in high stricture of esophagus. J. Thoracic Surg. *18:*316–326 (June) 1949.
14. Hays, R. P., and Clark, D. A.: Nutrition in patients with total gastrectomy and a jejunal food pouch. Ann. Surg. *152:*864–870 (Nov.) 1960.
15. Henley, F. A.: The surgical treatment of the "post-gastrectomy" syndrome. The Medical Press *233:*318–323 (Apr. 6) 1955.
16. Hirschhorn, R. C.: The decompensated ureter: A new experimental procedure for restoration of function. J. Urol. *90:*256–275 (Sept.) 1963.
17. Jordan, G. L., Jr., Angel, R. T., McIlhaney, J. S., Jr., et al.: Treatment of the post-gastrectomy dumping syndrome with a reversed jejunal segment interposed between the gastric remnant and the jejunum. Am. J. Surg. *106:*451–459 (Sept.) 1963.
18. Kasai, M., Abo, S., Makino, K., et al.: Reconstruction of the cervical esophagus with a pedicled jejunal graft. Surg. Gynec. & Obst. *121:*102–106 (July) 1965.
19. Key, J. A., Kergin, F. G., Martineau, Y., et al.: Method of supplementing the coronary circulation by jejunal pedicle graft. J. Thoracic Surg. *28:*320–330 (Sept.) 1954.
20. Knox, W. G.: Use of a jejunal pouch in treating post-gastrectomy malnutrition. Ann. Surg. *161:*35–40 (Jan.) 1965.
21. Lawrence, W., Jr., Kim, M., Isaacs, M., et al.: Gastric reservoir construction for severe disability after subtotal gastrectomy. Surg. Gynec. & Obst. *119:*1219–1232 (Dec.) 1964.
22. Lillehei, R. C. : Intestinal factor of irreversible hemorrhagic shock. Surgery *42:*1043–1054 (Dec.) 1957.
23. Lillehei, R. C., Goldberg, S., Goott, B., et al.: The present status of intestinal transplantation. Am. J. Surg. *105:*58–72 (Jan.) 1963.
24. Lillehei, R. C., Goott, B., and Miller, F. A.: The physiological response of the small bowel of the dog to ischemia including prolonged in vitro preservation of the bowel with successful replacement and survival. Ann. Surg. *150:*543–560 (Oct.) 1959.
25. Melnikoff, A. E.: Sur le remplacement de l'uretère par une anse isolée de l'intestine grêle. Rev. clin. d'urol. Par., *1:*601–613, 1912.
26. Moore, E. V., Weber, R., Woodward, E. R., et al.: Isolated ileal loops for ureteral repair. Surg. Gynec. & Obst. *102:*87–97 (Jan.) 1956.

27. Nakayama, K., Yamamoto, K., Tamiya, T., et al.: Experience with free autografts of the bowel with a new venous anastomosis apparatus. Surgery *55:*796–802 (June) 1964.
28. Poth, E. J.: Surgical correction of severe "dumping" and post-gastrectomy malnutrition: a therapeutic and diagnostic test. Ann. Surg. *160:*488–496 (Sept.) 1964.
29. Pyrah, L. N.: Use of segments of small and large intestine in urological surgery, with special reference to problem of ureterocolic anastomosis. J. Urol. *78:*683–720 (Dec.) 1957.
30. Roberts, R. E., and Douglass, F. M.: Replacement of the cervical esophagus and hypopharynx by a revascularized free jejunal autograft. Report of a case successfully treated. New England J. Med. *264:*342–344 (Feb. 16) 1961.
31. Rutledge, R. H.: Comments on Henley's remedial operation for dumping syndrome. Surgery *55:*762–768 (June) 1964.
32. Seidenberg, B., Rosenak, S. S., Hurwitt, E. S., et al.: Immediate reconstruction of the cervical esophagus by a revascularized isolated jejunal segment. Ann. Surg. *149:*162–171 (Feb.) 1959.
33. Shoemaker, W. C.: Reversed seromuscular grafts in urinary tract reconstruction. J. Urol. *74:*453–475 (Oct.) 1955.
34. Tasker, J. H.: Ileo-cystoplasty: A new technique; an experimental study with report of a case. Brit. J. Urol. *25:*349–357 (Dec.) 1953.
35. Torbey, K., and Waddell, W. R.: Function of the colon after removal of anal sphincters and replacement by denervated ileal segments. An experimental study. Ann. Surg. *154:*424–431 (Sept.) 1961.
36. Yudin, S. S.: The surgical construction of 80 cases of artificial esophagus. Surg. Gynec. & Obst. *78:*561–583 (June) 1944.

Chapter Seventeen

NONPEPTIC ULCERS

Occasionally, ulceration of the small intestine occurs unrelated to acid-pepsin, tumor, infectious process, regional enteritis, or mechanical abnormality. Since 1795, when Baillie[3] first mentioned this condition, the cause has been unknown. In 1948, Evert et al.[8] collected 130 cases of which 80 involved the ileum. A review in 1963 raised the total of known cases to only 170.[15]

Undoubtedly a few of these lesions were peptic ulcerations, lately attributed to the Zollinger-Ellison syndrome.[16] Until 1964, writers on this subject, when considering the etiology, listed possible causes as being related to vascular or neurologic disease, hormonal or nutritional influences, infections, and trauma.[11]

POTASSIUM CHLORIDE ULCERS

A marked increase in the incidence of nonspecific ulcer led Lindholmer et al.[13] and Baker et al.[4] in 1964 to review their experience with this condition. After this review they suggested a causative relationship between these ulcers and the oral administration of thiazide diuretics and enteric-coated potassium chloride. Because of the obvious importance of this drug-related etiology, a cooperative survey of 440 hospitals in this country and abroad was made by the pharmaceutical industry and the Food and Drug Administration.[12] Four hundred eighty-four cases were collected, of which 57 percent had received diuretics or potassium chloride. Enteric-coated potassium chloride was the most commonly used drug in these patients, and in a companion study in monkeys, potassium chloride given orally reproduced the lesions. It was concluded therefore that potassium chloride was a causative agent in some cases. It has been suggested from laboratory observations that as little as 0.5 to 1.0 gm. of potassium chloride can produce the typical circumferential ulceration.[6] Boley, Schultz, et al.[6] and Allen et al.[2] suggested

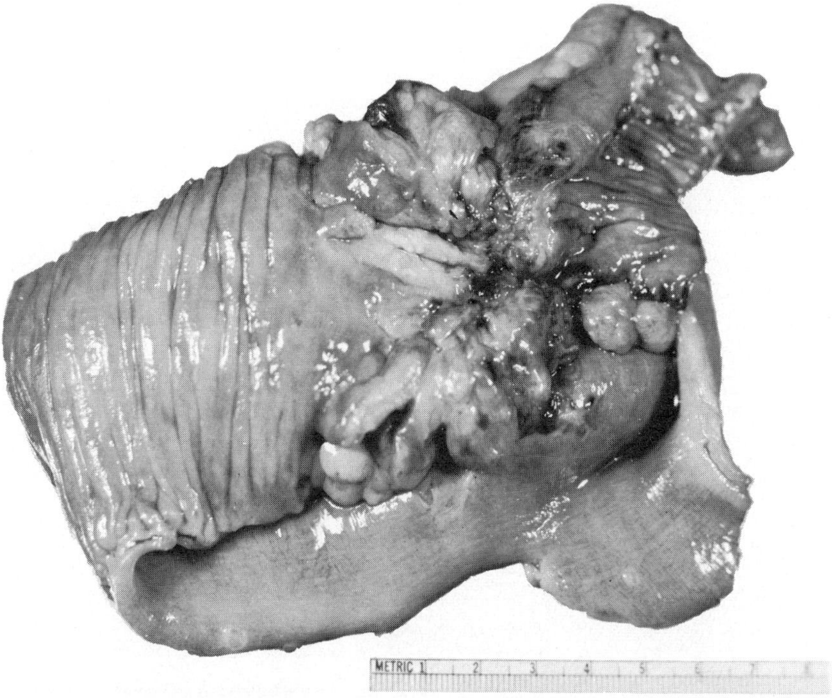

Figure 17-1. Typical circumferential ulcer of small intestine. Note dilated, obstructed proximal bowel and normal distal intestine (to right).

that this drug caused in sequence, venous spasm and stasis, submucosal edema, hemorrhagic segmental infarction, ulceration, and stenosis.

The symptoms of potassium chloride small bowel ulcers are most commonly abdominal pain, nausea, vomiting, and intermittent fullness.[14] The pain is most frequently postprandial, is crampy in nature, and may recur at intervals of from days to months. Occasionally multiple recurrences end with a catastrophic perforation. Occasionally hemorrhage is seen.[5] Radiographic studies of the small intestine show localized areas of obstruction with variable proximal distention.

The ulcers related to potassium therapy are strikingly uniform[14] (Figs. 17-1 and 17-2). There is a circumferential, sharply limited mucosal ulceration overlying a zone of cicatricial narrowing (Fig. 17-3). The width of the ulcerated zone averages 1.0 cm. Occasionally the ulcers are multiple. When perforated, the defects are round and measure approximately 1.0 cm. in diameter.

The treatment of these lesions has usually been resection with end-to-end anastomosis. The immediate results of this therapy have been excellent in spite of a resumption of chlorothiazide and potassium therapy in 6 of 17 cases reported by Morgenstern.[14] It is probable that earlier phases of the

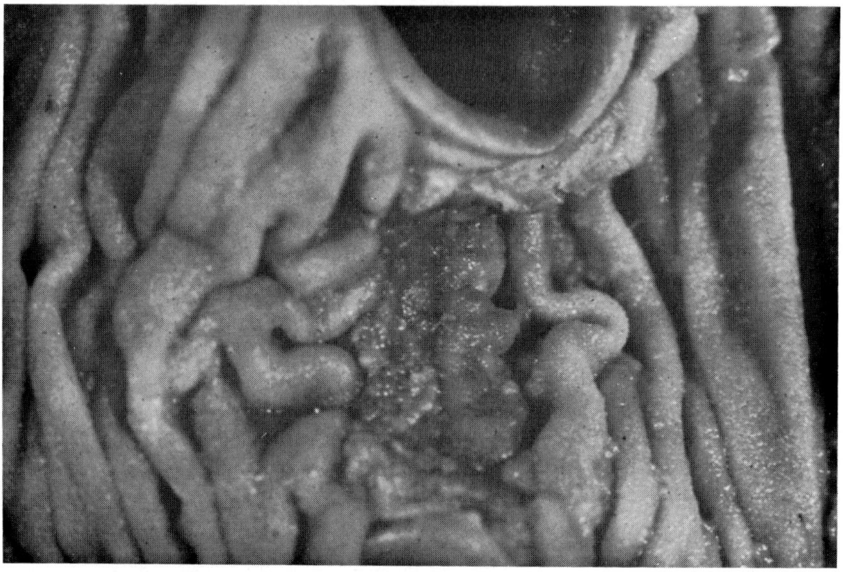

Figure 17–2. Close-up view of small bowel ulcer. (Courtesy of C. R. Hitchcock, M.D.)

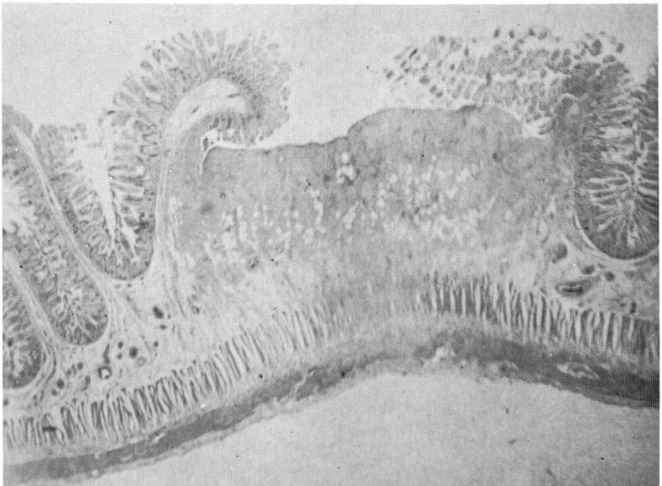

Figure 17–3. Cross section of small bowel ulcer (low power). Note sharply limited ulceration and submucosal increase in fibrous tissue. (Courtesy of C. R. Hitchcock, M.D.)

development of these ulcers will be recognized in the future. Therefore, if any unusual gastrointestinal symptoms develop in patients receiving potassium chloride with or without thiazides, the administration of the potassium chloride should be discontinued.[12] A case with reversible symptoms has been reported.[1] If the symptoms persist or recur, laparotomy and resection should be undertaken.[5]

NONSPECIFIC ULCERS

The nonspecific ulcers of the earlier literature are described as isolated and discrete in appearance with no surrounding inflammation.[10, 11] This type of ulcer involves the ileum twice as frequently as the jejunum and is usually single but sometimes occurs in small groups. Often it is located on the antimesenteric border of the intestine,[11] but other reports describe the nonpotassium ulcers as being circumferential also.[7]

The symptomatology of the nonspecific ulcer is similar to the circumferential ulcer in that there may be inflammation, perforation, hemorrhage or obstruction.[11] It has been suggested that the pain of this ulcer is not related to food intake,[8] whereas it is definitely postprandial in cases of circumferential ulcer.[14]

The treatment of this condition is generally resective, especially for perforation or hemorrhage, and the result should be satisfactory. A report of 20 patients who underwent resectional therapy and who were followed for a period from 1½ to 25 years revealed 13 to be asymptomatic.[9] Six had occasional mild discomfort and one had symptoms which might have been due to recurrent ulceration.

REFERENCES

1. Abbruzzese, A. A., and Gooding, C. A.: Reversible small-bowel obstruction: withdrawal of hydrochlorothiazide-potassium chloride therapy. J.A.M.A. *192:*781–782 (May 31) 1965.
2. Allen, A. C., Boley, S. J., Schultz, L., et al.: Potassium-induced lesions of the small bowel. II. Pathology and pathogenesis. J.A.M.A. *193:*1001–1006 (Sept. 20) 1965.
3. Baillie, M.: The Morbid Anatomy of Some of the Most Important Parts of the Human Body. The First American Edition. Albany, printed by Barker and Southwick, for Thomas Spencer, Bookseller, Market Street, 1795.
4. Baker, D. R., Schrader, W. H., and Hitchcock, C. R.: Small-bowel ulceration apparently associated with thiazide and potassium therapy. J.A.M.A. *190:*586–590 (Nov. 16) 1964.
5. Boley, S. J., Allen, A. C., Schultz, L., et al: Potassium-induced lesions of the small bowel. I. Clinical aspects, J.A.M.A. *193:*997–1000 (Sept. 20) 1965.
6. Boley, S. J., Schultz, L., Krieger, H., et al.: Experimental evaluation of thiazides and potassium as a cause of small-bowel ulcer. J.A.M.A. *192:*763–768 (May 31) 1965.
7. Brown, C. H., and Akin, N.: Stenosing small-intestinal ulcers; report of eleven cases. Cleveland Clin. Quart. *33:*85–93 (Apr.) 1966.

8. Evert, J. A., Black, B. M., and Dockerty, M. B.: Primary nonspecific ulcers of small intestine. Surgery *23:*185–200 (Feb.) 1948.
9. Goehrs, H. R., Morlock, C. G., and Dockerty, M. B.: Primary nonspecific ulcers of the small intestine. Proc. Staff Meet. Mayo Clin. *32:*351–353 (July 10) 1957.
10. Grasmann, M.: Ulcers of small intestine. Arch. klin. Chir. *136:*449–478, 1925.
11. Guest, J. L., Jr.: Nonspecific ulceration of the intestine. Internat. Abstr. Surg. *117:*409–416 (Nov.) 1963.
12. Lawrason, F. D., Alpert, E., Mohr, F. L., et al.: Ulcerative-obstructive lesions of the small intestine. J.A.M.A. *191:*641–644 (Feb. 22) 1965.
13. Lindholmer, B., Nyman, E., and Räf, L.: Nonspecific stenosing ulceration of the small bowel: a preliminary report. Acta chir. scandinav. *128:*310–311 (Sept.) 1964.
14. Morgenstern, L., Freilich, M., and Panish, J. F.: The circumferential small-bowel ulcer: clinical aspects in 17 patients. J.A.M.A. *191:*637–640 (Feb. 22) 1965.
15. Watson, M. R.: Primary nonspecific ulceration of the small bowel. Arch. Surg. *87:*600–603 (Oct.) 1963.
16. Zollinger, R. M., and Ellison, E. H.: Primary peptic ulcerations of jejunum associated with islet cell tumors of pancreas. Ann. Surg. *142:*709–728 (Oct.) 1955.

Chapter Eighteen

PNEUMATOSIS CYSTOIDES INTESTINALIS

This rare condition is characterized by the presence of gas-filled cysts in the wall and mesentery of the gastrointestinal tract. A condition with identical morphology is found also in hogs.[6] Pseudonyms include pneumatosis intestinalis, pneumatosis, gas cysts of the intestine, intestinal emphysema, and bullous emphysema of the intestine. According to Koss,[3] these lesions were first described by John Duvernoy[2] in the eighteenth century. An extensive review of the literature in 1952 disclosed 255 reported cases.[3]

Pneumatosis is seen at all ages and may be found throughout the abdominal intestinal tract, but it occurs most commonly in middle age in males and in the sixth decade in women.[8] Its distribution is subserosal or occasionally submucosal in the proximal jejunum, ileocecal area, and colon in descending frequency. At times, other intraabdominal structures are also involved. The cysts vary from microscopic size to several centimeters in diameter.

Fifteen percent of cases have no other disease, but 85 percent are associated with other lesions of the gastrointestinal tract, the most common of which is pyloric stenosis due to peptic ulcer.[3] In addition, other inflammatory intestinal lesions or diarrheal states such as diverticulitis have been associated.

There is no evidence that is helpful in establishing the etiology of this condition. Gas analysis reveals the contents to be composed of about 90 percent nitrogen, 8 percent carbon dioxide and 2 percent oxygen.[5] Careful inspection of the mucosal lining of the involved bowel has failed to disclose breaks in the mucous membrane that would permit gas to pass from the bowel lumen into the tissues. There is no evidence of infection in or around the cysts on a microscopic or bacteriologic basis nor anything from a clinical standpoint to suggest a role played by bacteria.[4, 7] Chronic pulmonary disease

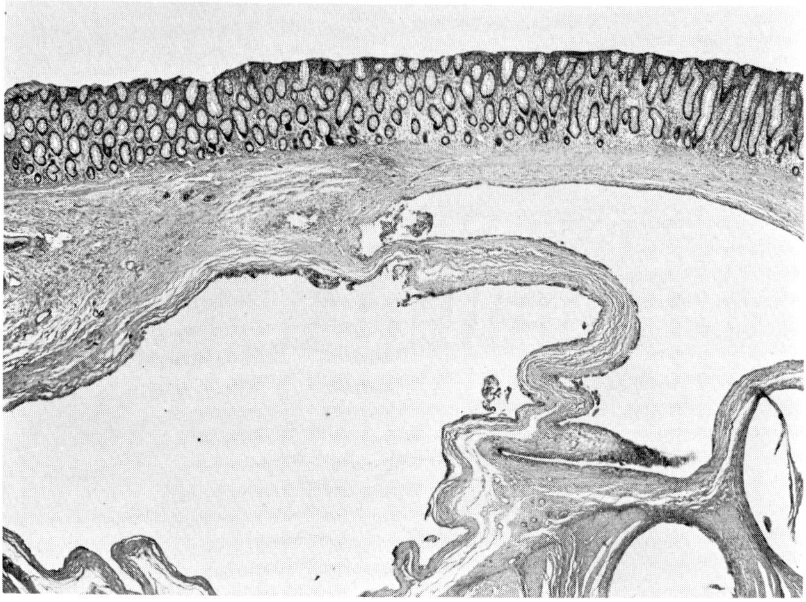

Figure 18–1. Photomicrograph of pneumatosis intestinalis.

has been implicated as a causative factor in some cases. Since a high proportion of cases are associated with pyloric stenosis or intestinal obstruction, an increase in intraluminal pressure has been thought to be responsible for this lesion. Microscopic examination (Fig. 18–1) usually reveals no well-defined lining membrane around the gas spaces, but occasionally a flat endothelium may be present. Druckmann et al.[1] believe that in adults pneumatosis follows malnutrition and that when this is relieved the pneumatosis disappears.

The symptoms of this condition are variable and are probably those of the underlying disease. Occasionally hemorrhage from obstruction of involved segments is seen. The obstruction may be due to external compression of the bowel or direct obstruction of the lumen. In addition, volvulus and intussusception secondary to the cysts have been reported.[3] Cases of malabsorption due to extensive pneumatosis[9] and of tension pneumoperitoneum from rupture of the cysts have been encountered.[3]

The diagnosis of the disease is made at autopsy, at surgery, or on plain or contrast examination of the abdomen or intestine. Radiolucent areas occurring in clusters that follow the contour of the bowel are diagnostic. The finding of pneumoperitoneum without a ruptured viscus is suggestive and illustrates one of the complications of the condition. Gas present in the mesenteric and retroperitoneal planes is also suggestive.

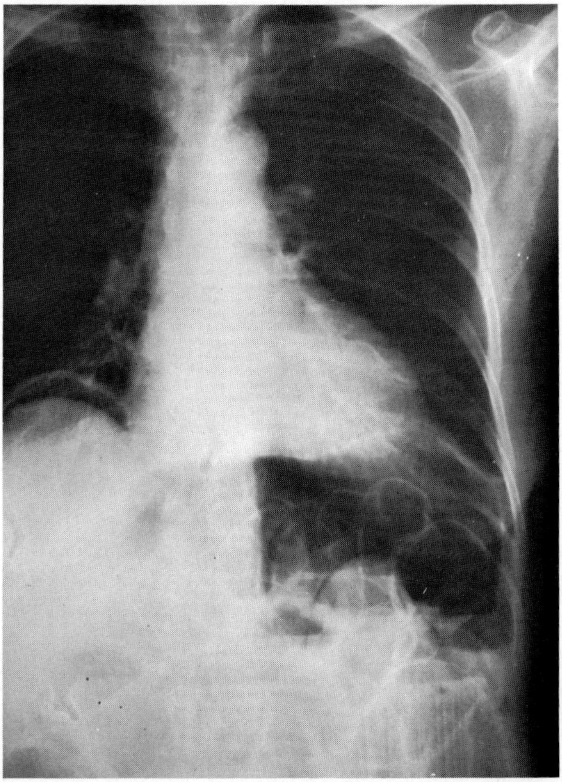

Figure 18–2. Roentgenogram of abdomen showing free air under right diaphragm and gas cysts in left upper quadrant.

CASE REPORT

A 67-year-old female was admitted to the hospital complaining of left lower quadrant abdominal discomfort and a "pressure feeling" throughout her abdomen. Six months previously she had noted the onset of diarrhea with generalized abdominal cramping associated initially with a fever of 101°. The diarrhea persisted, but her temperature returned to normal after one or two days. A few days before admission she noticed progressive abdominal distention.

Seven years before admission she had had a cholecystectomy, and three years before admission the diagnosis of gout was made. Previous barium enemas had shown sigmoid diverticulosis.

On examination there was moderate distention of the abdomen without much tenderness or rigidity. The abdomen was tympanitic, and bowel sounds were frequent. She passed gas per rectum. The temperature was normal, as were the following blood tests: hemoglobin, white count, differential count, alkaline phosphatase, proteins, urea, chloride, sodium, potassium, calcium, and phosphorus.

A roentgenogram of the abdomen showed free air under the diaphragm, distention of the bowel, and a peculiar appearance of the small bowel loops in the left upper quadrant (Fig. 18–2).

Because of the possibility of a ruptured viscus, laparotomy was performed. The small intestine and its mesentery were involved with a myriad of cysts measuring from a few millimeters to several centimeters in diameter. There was no odor from the peritoneal cavity and no inflammation of the peritoneum.

Comment. This case is typical of pneumatosis, the indication for surgery being a suspected ruptured viscus.

The treatment of this condition is almost always that of the associated disease. Rarely, hemorrhage or obstruction demand resection of the involved small intestine.

REFERENCES

1. Druckmann, A., Schwartz, A., Rabinovici, N., et al.: Pneumatosis of the intestines. Am. J. Roentgenol. *86:*911–919 (Nov.) 1961.
2. Duvernoy, J. G.: cited by Combalusier: Pneumopathologie ou traité des maladies venteuses. Paris, 1754, 1, 19.
3. Koss, L. G.: Abdominal gas cysts (pneumatosis cystoides intestinorum hominis); analysis with report of case and critical review of literature. Arch. Path. *53:*523–549 (June) 1952.
4. Moore, R. A.: Intestinal pneumatosis. Am. J. Dis. Child. *38:*818–823 (Oct.) 1929.
5. Mujahed, Z., and Evans, J. A.: Gas cysts of the intestine (pneumatosis intestinalis). Surg. Gynec. & Obst. *107:*151–160 (Aug.) 1958.
6. Nitch, C. A. R.: Cystic pneumatosis of intestinal tract. Brit. J. Surg. *11:*714–736 (Apr.) 1924.
7. Silverstone, J.: Case of cystic pneumatosis of bowel. Lancet *1:*129–130 (Jan. 21) 1928.
8. Stiennon, O. A.: Pneumatosis intestinalis in the newborn. Am. J. Dis. Child. *81:*651–663 (May) 1951.
9. Yunich, A. M., and Fradkin, N. F.: Fatal sprue (malabsorption) syndrome secondary to extensive pneumatosis cystoides intestinalis. Gastroenterology *35:*212–217 (July) 1958.

Index

Italic page numbers refer to illustrations; those followed by (t) refer to tables.